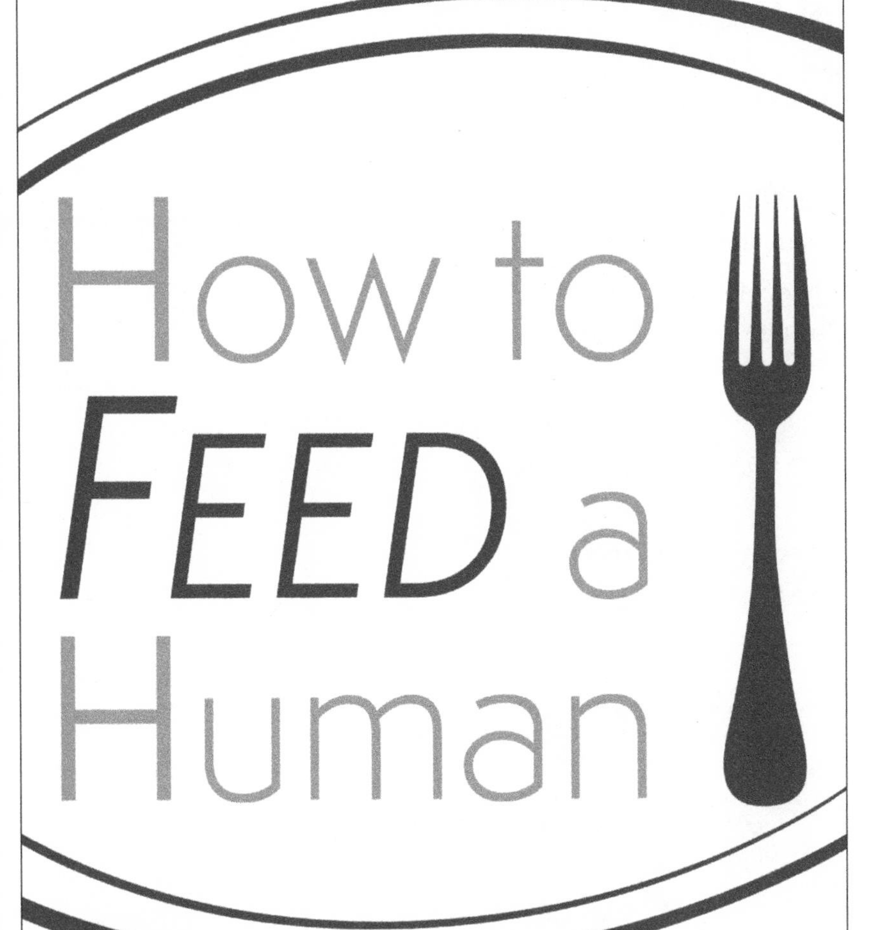

The
Whole Food Muscle
Way

How to Feed a Human The Whole Food Muscle Way
ISBN 978-0-9846581-2-1

Published by Champion Performance Development
www.ChampPerformance.com

Edited by Nancy LaFever
www.EditorChick.com

Cover Art by Russell Bruzzano
www.RgBDesignGroup.com

Book Layout and Design by Russell Bruzzano
www.RgBDesigngroup.com

Printed in the United States of America

Disclaimer

This book is designed to provide information in regard to the subject matter covered. It contains the opinions, ideas, advice and stories of its authors related to health, wellness, nutrition and fitness. It is intended to provide general information on those subjects and should be used as a supplement to, not in replacement of, advice from your doctor and other qualified medical professionals. Before changing your existing diet or fitness program or starting a new one it is recommended that you consult your personal physician. Additionally, it is wise to stay engaged with your physician throughout your health journey. Every effort has been made to assure the accuracy of the information contained in this book as of the date of publication. This book is sold or provided with the understanding that the publisher, authors, editor, and/or sponsor(s) shall not be held liable in any degree for any loss or injury due to any omission, error, misprinting, or ambiguity. The publisher, editor and the authors disclaim any personal liability, directly or indirectly, for any medical or personal outcomes that may occur as a result of applying the methods presented in this book.

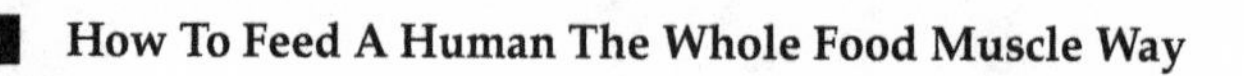

Foreword

Two competitive athletes, Dr Robyn (beach volleyball) and Russ (bodybuilding) personally experienced that they could not prevent the serious health conditions including weight gain that comes with eating the Standard American Diet despite a very rigorous daily exercise program. As Dr Robyn puts it "You can't out exercise a bad diet." Exceptional health starts and ends with the fuel we feed our bodies.

Dr Robyn thought she was healthy, but experienced weight gain and high cholesterol requiring statins despite working out 5 days/week and biking anywhere from 50-100 miles/week. Due to the painful side effects she experienced from the statin medication, she made a decision to find another solution. She ultimately discovered that the road to optimal health and vitality came with eating plants.

This book is an easy-to-follow journey of two competitive athletes who recount their evolution to discovering an ideal plan that anyone can use to reach their ideal weight and health goals.

The most common complaint I hear from many of my female (and a few male) patients that have adopted a healthy plant-based lifestyle is that they cannot attain the weight goal they wish despite regular exercising and eliminating animal products and processed foods. They may have initially lost weight, but have now plateaued and cannot reach their goal weight.

This book holds the solution!

Dr Robyn and Russ have included, in my opinion, a surefire strategy which will solve this frustrating problem--intermittent fasting. They do a superb job of defining the concept, why it is so essential for our weight loss efforts, optimal health, and longevity, and how to easily incorporate it into our daily regimen.

This book is the superlative roadmap to being the best you can be!

Ted Crawford, D.O.
Board Certified Family Physician
Member of the American College of Lifestyle Medicine
Featured in the documentary "Eating You Alive"

Meet the Authors

Hi, I'm Dr Robyn. You'll find that most of this book is written in my voice because I did the typing. Russ has been an integral part of the content creation over untold conversations, drafts and rewrites. He is always my biggest cheerleader. The cover design and book layout are his vision and work.

Part of what makes us a great team is our individual backgrounds as competitive athletes and our willingness to allow each other to take the lead with our respective talents. Russ was a bodybuilder one level from going pro when he retired to travel Europe as a trainer on the Mr. Olympia tour (Check out his profile at www.RnRJourney.com/about to see a picture from back in the day). And I spent more weekends than I can count on the sand playing beach volleyball. Both of us have moved beyond our competition days, but you will still find us working out a minimum of five days a week in the gym and riding our hybrid bikes as many miles as we can squeeze in. Our athletic pasts are reflected in the exercise component of the Whole Food Muscle™ Way with exercise plans and suggestions by Russ. When was the last time you had a Mr. Olympia trainer create a workout for you?

Together Russ and I have spent thousands of hours reading, studying, taking classes and discussing nutrition and longevity science and the research on intermittent fasting. I earned the certificate from the Center for Nutrition Studies at Cornell University because I enjoy academic rigor, whereas Russ is more practical, wanting to jump right into applying the science to real life.

Throughout this book you'll find that is a recurring theme. We always strive to create a balance between science and real-life application.

You will also find that my background in psychology, including sport psychology, and my years as an executive coach play an active role in the Whole Food Muscle Way. Self-sabotage, other-sabotage, emotional eating and eating out of habit are all realities that could derail your desire to create and maintain a healthy lifestyle. I address those challenges and provide practical tips you can use right away to address them.

Finally, I would be remiss if I didn't warn you. This book and the Whole Food Muscle Way are not for people looking for a quick fix, easy way out or an excuse to fail. We created this system and wrote this book for people who want to succeed and who are willing to take the steps necessary to do so. Our goal is to provide you with an effective, proven, step-by-step method in an easy-to-apply manner. Those who have worked with us say we provide inspiration and motivation in a knowledgeable, nonjudgmental, relatable, no-nonsense way. Think of us like your sports coach. We love you, believe in you and want to you succeed. And as such, we are going to tell you the hard truths and call you out on your nonsense while celebrating every single one of your accomplishments.

If that sounds like a path you can follow to success, let's get started.

We'll see you on the inside.

Contents

Contents continued

We are excited to be part of your health journey!

Let's Jump Right In

Introduction

Every high performance, elite success and peak achievement book has a line or a paragraph that says something like, "Physical health is the foundation of accomplishment. Eat well, get some exercise and get enough sleep." Some might even go on to give you tips on how to fit more sleep and exercise into your life. They all just assume you know how to "eat well." But based on the surging rates of obesity, diabetes, heart disease, high blood pressure and high cholesterol, it's clear that even those at the top of their success rarely know anything about the nutrition they are putting through their bodies.

But it's not your fault. We have been programmed (by the food industry and other entities we will discuss throughout this book) to believe that nutrition is confusing and time-consuming.

For example, the food industry has convinced us through slick marketing campaigns that we need fast, convenient calories so we can "get on with" our busy lives. We have been tricked into believing food must equal pleasure; if we aren't in ecstasy with every bite, we are somehow missing out on something. Those ideas come from marketing messages designed to make big corporations money. They certainly don't have our best interest or health in mind.

There is a certain type of person who has the willingness and ability to see through the marketing and realize that their very lives are at stake. A few have the desire to do something about it. They are the high achievers. They decide what they want and go after it 100%. Their goal is to reach the top and to stay there. You must be one of us because you are reading this book.

Then there are those who are happy with the status quo, who let life live them and who don't care about gaining an edge on the competition. They are happy going through life being told what to do and when to do it by someone else.

Take a look at your eating habits. Wow, what a letdown. What happened? Why are you powering through each day everyday doing amazing things in so many areas of your life, but the one thing that makes sure you have the energy and stamina to keep climbing – the food you eat – you treat like an afterthought if you think about it at all?

I can tell you why. Because the nutrition advice we hear *is* confusing. What's good for us or bad for us seems to change on a daily basis. The "science" (we'll discuss why that's in quotes later) we hear seems to conflict and contradict itself every other day. Unless you have time to trudge through books, articles, journals, lectures and classes every time another study hits the press (and clearly you don't), it is nearly impossible to know and keep up with the truth. So, you do the best you can and hope it's good enough.

I can tell you why else what you eat is an afterthought. It's because it is easier to choose short-term pleasure and gratification over your long-term goals. Don't bristle about that. Deep down you know it's true. You don't WANT to have to think about what you eat. You don't like veggies. You WANT to eat pizza and beer and steak and burgers, and, and, and… Self-gratification much?

In your twenties and maybe into your thirties, that was acceptable and "good enough." It's not anymore. Your body is starting to crack under the strain. You're soft around the middle (okay, likely more than "soft"). Maybe you're on a medication, or two, or three. Your doctor (assuming you go) has suggested you take better care of yourself. And your inner voice says, "Yeah,

I need to" and you think about going on a diet next week. That lasts until you open your email and you're back into the grind that is your life where your health and body are given a backseat on a joyride that is getting more and more dangerous.

But you aren't the kind of person to sit back and let things happen around you. You are a person of action. Once you know what needs to be done, you do it with gusto.

That starts for your health now.

Look, you don't have to be a nutritionist or have a PhD in biochemistry to understand, apply and benefit from the ideas in this book. The complex research, development and testing have already been done for you. We have spent thousands of hours slogging through the science, books, lectures, classes and conflicting information about how nutrition, motivation, self-discipline and cultural pressure apply to health, longevity and elite success. We've condensed the results into this simple, but powerful guide anyone can use to motivate themselves to achieve their life goals and dreams while enjoying the journey. We call it The Whole Food Muscle Way.

We have broken your optimum performance into three easy-to-apply ideas.

- Being sick and unhealthy has become the norm and taking care of your body gets you labeled a "health nut." But you aren't 100% to blame for being so far off track. We have been sold a bill of goods that is killing us. After reading these few pages, you'll be able to spot the ruse and stop making unconscious choices about your health.

- If what you are eating is made in a plant, comes in a ready-to-eat package or is designed to make a corporation money, you can be sure it was not made with your health and vitality in mind. It's not your fault that companies have twisted the "science" to say what they want it to say and advertise and market it as they see fit. It's also not your fault that those same companies use the money they make from their in-house science to create government policy that allows them to continue to trick and confuse us. It is, however, your responsibility to learn the truth and take care of yourself and those you love.

- We systematically guide you through how to integrate your new-found knowledge into your life. It doesn't do you any good to know the principles if it doesn't change what goes into your stomach. You'll also learn how to spot and overcome common pitfalls to your success, such as Pavlovian eating, emotional eating, the feeling you're missing out and peer pressure (you wouldn't think that would be a thing at this point in your life, but it is. And it's a bigger thing than you realize).

Most people aren't healthy because they have never really experienced what it is like to have a body that hums along like a well-oiled machine. They don't know, or don't remember, what they are missing. Once you create good health, you'll be hooked on it and wonder how you ever functioned in your current sluggish, overweight, lethargic state.

You're about to learn, once and for all, that the food you choose to eat is the master key to your success. Not only are you going to know why, but you'll have an in-depth understanding of the choices you have been letting someone else make for you. You have fought hard to succeed forcing yourself through, over and around challenges with grit and determination. Now there is a tiny voice in your head that fears you are falling behind and are on the verge of catastrophically failing. It's time to wrestle back control and enjoy the vibrant ease that comes with reaching and maintaining the success that most people envy, but consider out of reach.

We have done it. And in the short time it takes you to read this book, so will you.

Note: This book is not meant to be an academic dive into the research that supports this way of eating as the optimal diet and nutrition for human health and longevity. There are MANY already on the market. If you're interested in the source materials and science, visit *www.RnRJourney.com/resources* for a list of books we recommend.

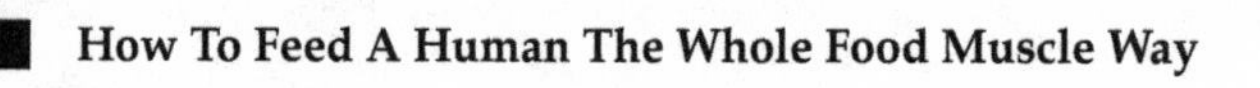

What We've Been Told Isn't Working

Looking through our notes from the onboarding meeting with a new executive client we had to be impressed. He had a remarkable resumé of accomplishments and awards to his credit. And he was able to easily articulate his short-, mid- and long-term goals. He had an idea of where he had some work to do and he was clear on why he chose to work with us. He had laughed, "I need someone who will stand up to me, tell me when I'm missing something… make me think. You do that just sitting at dinner."

We had met a few weeks earlier at a corporate event where we had enjoyed being seated at a table with eight other people who actually wanted to have conversations. No one just pontificated while everyone else had to eat in silence and listen. It had been a fun evening of sharing ideas and banter.

I smiled. *"In that vein, let's talk about your priorities."*

He rattled off about half a dozen work-related topics.

"Are those in order of importance?"

He gave a little shrug. *"Mostly. Depends on what's on fire."*

We chuckled. Yeah. That's life. It's hard to work on what's important when there is always something urgent demanding your attention.

(**Side note:** This is how most people treat their bodies and their health, they only work on something if it is "on fire" and needs urgent attention. In this book, you'll discover a better approach.)

"What about personally?" I prodded.

"What do you mean?" He looked confused.

"How do your personal plans and priorities fit in here?"

"You mean like retirement?"

No matter how often it happens (and it's quite often), it always surprises us when a successful, high-powered, peak performer at the top of their game becomes confused when we want to talk about more than spreadsheets, metrics and managing people.

"If that's in your five-year plan, yes, but your day-to-day family, social and personal well-being...?" I raised an eyebrow.

He huffed. People, especially high performers, always hate this part of the conversation. Heaven forbid they look at themselves personally.

It took some good-natured prodding but he admitted with a grudging laugh, that yes, his wife and three kids were important and needed to be on the list.

"What about your health?"

"Yeah…" his voice trailed off as he drew his mouth into a tight, downturned line.

My experience as a high-performance coach and our expertise in health and longevity nutrition and exercise were why he was working with us. But they weren't topics he enjoyed thinking about.

We have been lied to and we believe it

There are 500,000 open heart surgeries performed every year. The idea of having your chest cracked open, your ribs torqued back and a vein from your leg tacked on your heart has become commonplace (think about that for a minute). So common, in fact, the past president of the American Heart Association, Timothy Gardner says, *"It's a very safe operation."* Considering that the death rate before being discharged is between 1 and 3% (that's between 5,000 and 15,000 people a year for those counting), we guess that's pretty safe. But really? Normal? Particularly when it's known that heart disease is caused by and can be reversed by diet and up to 40% of bypasses close up within a year? Are we really that self-indulgent and love fat, salt and sugar that much? Yes, it seems we do.

But the Standard American Diet (SAD), also called the Western Diet, isn't just causing heart disease. We can blame diabetes, high blood pressure, high cholesterol and obesity squarely on it as well. If all of these diseases are diet-related, why isn't something being done about it?

That is a very astute question.

How living sick became the norm

Your health is big business. Actually, your sickness is big business. Healthy people don't run up big medical bills. The medical system was set up to find treatments that could be patented and sold. You can't get a patent for telling people to eat vegetables. But take a compound out of a vegetable, synthesize it, put it in pill form and voilà! You have something you can patent, market and profit from. And if you call it a "supplement," you don't even need FDA approval to sell it.

And profit they do! How many drug commercials have you seen in the last week? If you watch any TV at all, probably too many to remember. Big Pharma takes medical students out to fancy dinners. Why? Because they know doctors can be turned into pill pushers. Have a problem? No worries, you can just pop a pill for that. And it doesn't stop when they get out of school. Pharma rep is a real job. They go from doctor to doctor bringing unhealthy lunches and drug samples to make sure the pill pushers know about their pill.

You might think we are being overly dramatic. But doctors spend thousands of hours studying what pills treat what disease. And when we say "treat," we don't necessarily mean "cure." Many drugs are just meant to moderate symptoms, not actually fix the problem. That's fancy talk for, "You'll be on this pill for the rest of your life." Cha-ching!

> ***The idea of having your chest cracked open, your ribs torqued back and a vein from your leg tacked on your heart has become commonplace.***

Care to guess how much time doctors spend learning about how nutrition relates to health, disease and longevity? Don't guess.

We'll tell you – typically less than 30 hours and many get zero.

Unless they go out of their way on their own time to research and study nutrition, they know as much as you could learn about an incredibly complicated job in one, part-time work week. And the classes they do take are usually focused on the biology and biochemistry of how the body processes food, not on how the lack of nutrients or way too many nutrients make us sick.

Consider this – when was the last time you saw a doctor who you would describe as being healthy and at their ideal weight?

Now, we aren't saying doctors are evil, out to get you or consciously trying to keep you sick.

Doctors absolutely have their place and advances in modern medicine are amazing.

However, we are saying that doctors don't know what they don't know. And they are so enveloped in sickness care that they can't hear the truth about nutrition. As a high-performer, you know that to keep your edge, you HAVE to be willing to educate yourself so you can make critical decisions based on facts.

We don't have to tell you that. That's why you're holding this book.

There's big money in what you eat!

When food companies convinced us that cooking and feeding ourselves were mundane chores that no one had time for, they tapped into a never-ending stream of income and their stockholders have been doing happy dances all the way to the bank since. But at what cost?

We have outsourced the thing our body needs most next to oxygen and water – nutrition.

Nutrition is, after all, the essential ingredient that gives your body energy, allows it to fight disease and keeps all your trillions of cells humming along doing their thing. We're letting profit-driven corporate conglomerates tell us what to eat because we "don't have time." About now your brain should be screaming at you, "That's a problem!"

There have been attempts to get Big Food to own up to its role in the health and obesity crisis in this country. But they just say, "We aren't anybody's nanny. We aren't telling anyone they have to eat our stuff. We're not suggesting people eat it all the time. It's just for a snack for when they're in a hurry or, or, or…" So many excuses for why their profit-generating junk is just fine and our health is not their problem.

But in the meantime, Big Food is spending millions of dollars on research to find out how to perfectly trick your body into thinking what they are selling is food. Package coloring that millions of years of evolution tells your Caveman Brain, "Hey this is the healthiest fruit with the most nutrients."

Never mind that what is actually in the package is processed plant fragments with chemical flavoring and zero nutritional value. Plus, the millions more dollars being spent to tease your taste buds with "flavor" that overrides your "I've had enough" switch so you keep eating, even when you're not hungry (more eating = more profits, so eat up!)

Big Food employs expensive lobbyists who convince Congress they just make the offering, you make the choice. You can choose not to eat it if you want. But can you really? Based on the visceral response we get when we even so much as suggest people give up cheese, you don't have a choice. You're addicted to the fat, sugar and salt laden "food" being pumped full of synthesized flavor by the food industry.

That's not very high performance of you, is it?

"Science" isn't science at all

One of our favorite (when we say "favorite," we mean eye-rollingly ridiculous) studies (when we say "studies" we mean, "industry-funded nonsense passed off as science") is where the egg industry showed that eating eggs doesn't raise cholesterol.

Here's how that works (spoiler, it's not true):

The human body can only absorb so much cholesterol. There comes a point where it just maxes out. If you have people eat enough cholesterol-rich food (found in animal products), their cholesterol reading will max out. At that point they can eat an egg or ten and their cholesterol reading won't go up. That is how maxing something out works. But, do it in a research lab and release the results to the press with a conveniently worded abstract and suddenly every major paper and morning talk show is saying eggs don't raise cholesterol.

Shady? Yep. Illegal? Nope.

If you Google the definition of the word "science" you will see something along the lines of: "Facts, knowledge or principles gathered through systematic study, observation or experimentation." That seems pretty straight forward. BUT that definition doesn't say anything about being unbiased, testing an actual theory, using reasonable statistic methods, rigging study results to line up with corporate profit goals or any other manipulation insuring the "facts" shared with the public are actually universally true. The beverage industry does it by conveniently leaving water out of their experiments (Drinking soda is better than dying of dehydration!).

There is also no legal definition of what does or does not constitute science. You could stand outside your office and count how many redheads walk by in a certain time frame, run some fancy stats and predict how many redheads live in the world. It's unlikely to be valid. But don't let that little issue worry you. It's science!

The vast majority of what is touted as science comes from one of two places, the academic world or directly from the food and drug industries. We can write off the food and drug industry science as biased without much thought. They are openly trying to make money and looking for results that will sell product. Why would they do a trial testing their latest drug against broccoli sprouts? Broccoli sprouts might win (actually, we would put money on it) and where would that leave them? You can't get a patent on broccoli sprouts, so there's no money to be made!

But what about academic research? Research requires funding. And the people/corporations who fund studies want outcomes they can use to make a profit. If you had the time and the desire to dig into nutrition science, you'd find that most of it is funded by industry. Even the nonprofits that provide funding have corporate donors they need to appease. A researcher's reputation and career can be ruined if they somehow manage to get funding and publish results that make industry look bad. So, no. Academic research isn't unbiased either.

And let's not forget the issue of publication bias. This is the act of only publishing studies that show what they want the public to know and hiding everything else in a filing cabinet in an offsite storage unit.

It may seem far-fetched, that someone would hide their research because they didn't like the results, but it happens in "science" all the time.

Don't worry. We aren't going to leave you floating in this morass of unknown forever. But, while we're at it, let's talk about the diet industry.

Diets, diets and more diets

The diet industry has been estimated to be worth as high as 80 billion dollars a year. That is A LOT of people trying to lose weight. But diets fail to produce sustainable results 98% of the time. It's the same 60-80% of the population losing 20 pounds and gaining back 30, over and over until they just give up.

Diets are only about losing weight. That is their only goal. Long-term health, nutrition and longevity aren't even on the to-do list. There are lots of ways to lose weight: heroin, cocaine, chemo, getting really sick, diet pills from the 1970s. No one (at least we hope no one) is going to choose any of those options on purpose because we know the damage to our health isn't worth it. And yet, when the newest fad diet shows up on the news, we somehow forget that a "quick fix" is NOT a good idea and we clamor on the bandwagon.

> *Big Food is spending millions of dollars on research to find out how to perfectly trick your body into thinking what they are selling is food.*

Some of the popular fads right now:

Low carb - People lose weight on low carb diets because they also tend to cut calories. It is impossible to sustain low calorie intake over the long-term. And since your body runs best on carbs, high fat/high protein intake gums up the inner workings. The science is clear, diets (whether we are "dieting" or not) high in fat and animal protein don't do a body good.

What about the argument: But our ancestors ate tons of meat during the Paleolithic Period? That study was never meant to inform how we should eat now. Early humans certainly weren't eating animal products three or more times a day seven days a week. Some estimates are as low as 3% of their diet was animal-based. And we couldn't eat like a Paleo-human if we tried. That food is just not available. And even if it were, eating like a Paleo-human is like feeding your dog based on what a stray is scavenging. Paleo-humans ate what they could find in hopes of staying alive long enough to procreate (which some did; fortunately for us). The optimal diet for health and longevity crossed their minds as often as they went to the grocery store (that, for the record, would be never). Not to mention, humans in the Paleolithic Period got more exercise than everyone in your office combined and didn't live long enough to get heart disease, diabetes, obesity, high blood pressure and high cholesterol.

Even if you don't cut calories, eating low-carb puts your body into survival mode. And yes, that will cause you to lose weight. Your body will literally eat itself. And that's not a good thing. There are consequences to your heart, kidneys, endothelium (the lining of your blood vessels that keeps gunk from sticking), cholesterol levels, blood pressure and overall health. It is an all-around horrible idea. Oh, and just for good measure, the weight loss results won't last, but the damage to your body will.

If low-carb was viable, we wouldn't have an obesity epidemic. The Adkins Diet was created in the 1960s. He died obese and with heart disease. We think five-ish decades of real-life human study is long enough to say it's clearly not working.

Shakes/delivered food - People lose weight on these diets because again, they cut calories from what they would normally eat. Unless you can see yourself buying that food and staying on that plan forever, it is not a long-term solution for weight loss. Not to mention our bodies are designed to chew food and eat until we are full. We are interested in the lifetime safety of items designed to trick our body into not chewing or being full. So far there is no longitudinal (long- term) data. The people taking them now can let us know in 20-30 years how it turned out for them.

Patches to boost metabolism - Stimulants aren't the choice we would make for our health. Anything that pushes the body's adrenals sounds like a short-term "fix" to a long-term problem. High performers don't look for the quick way; they look for the right way.

Whole nutrition in a capsule - Unless a company has created a Jetsons-type pill that contains all the vitamins, minerals, fiber, protein, carbohydrates, fat, calories, water and bulk that is in the real, whole plants, and can cause people to reach and maintain their ideal weight easily while improving their health, it's not whole-food. It is the extracted parts that some scientist deemed worthy of being included. If the package the nutrients came in (i.e., the whole fruit/veggie/legume) isn't there, "whole" isn't the right word. These products are considered "supplements," so there are no safety standards and these companies are self-policed. Why would you trust your health to the honesty of a corporation out to make a dollar when you could just get the perfect balance of nutrients you need from actual food?

This is the million-dollar question about pills, potions, lotions and lore: have they been put to the scientific test against a whole-food plant-based lifestyle (or at least something close)? That is the gold standard because humans have been doing pretty well on it for a LONG time AND all the recent science (the last 100 years or so) has found that eating plants is pretty darn good for us. Not to mention there is no need to count calories! But when you look into what is being offered as the supporting research for many of these diets and products (assuming they've done research), they aren't testing it against eating mostly plants. We are guessing that is because they know their product would lose and that would be bad for business!

If it was made in a plant, it's likely not food - Over the years there have been several "magic bullet" solutions provided by industry that were supposed to save us from metabolic diseases. Sadly, they are myths and have made things worse, not better. Here are three big ones:

Myth – Fake sweeteners will save us from obesity (see the chapter, **Artificial Sweeteners are Damaging Your Gut**)

Truth – Various fake sweeteners are associated with migraine risk, insulin resistance (which leads to diabetes), irritable bowel disease, and Crohn's disease. And just for good measure, because your body was expecting calories due to the sweetness and didn't get calories, it makes you eat more calories later than you otherwise would have. So, they don't help with the obesity issue, they make it worse.

What to do instead – Regular sugar isn't horrible for you. At least your body knows how to process it. The problem is the huge quantities of it in most people's diets due to eating processed food-like stuff. Sugar should be used sparingly and to encourage us to eat real, whole-plant foods or as a treat to be savored. Blackstrap molasses and date sugar (which is just dried dates and not really sugar) both have the same calories as sugar but they do have some nutritional value. We also use real maple syrup. No better for us than sugar. Just less processed.

Eat food your body recognizes as food.

Myth – Low fat will save us from heart disease

Truth – When we were told that fat was making us fat and killing us with heart disease, we listened and suddenly anything with "low-fat" splashed across the package became synonymous with "healthy" and we could eat as much of it as we wanted. Unfortunately, sugar (often fake sugar to keep the calories down) was typically added to make up for the lost flavor. And in the case of dairy products, reducing the fat content increased the percentage of unhealthy animal protein. Thirty + years on from the start of the low-fat craze, we are fatter and heart disease is killing more of us than ever.

What to do instead: The issue isn't "fat" across the board. It is the saturated fats found in animal-based products (meat, dairy, eggs) and processed plant fats (oil). Become a flexitarian (eating meat only once or maybe twice a week) and you reduce your risk of heart disease by 27%. Adopt a vegetarian diet (no meat) and you can drop your risk 53%. Go vegan (no meat, dairy or eggs) and your risk drops 61%. But what if you go whole-food plant-based, the Whole Food Muscle way of eating, (no meat, dairy or eggs, and minimize oils and sugar, AND eat high-fat plants like nuts)? Now your risk of dying of heart disease drops a striking 80%!

Myth – Eating carbs* is making us fat (see the chapter, **Carbs are Not the Devil**)

Truth – Whole-food carbohydrates are GOOD for us. They are what our bodies are designed to use as fuel to run our trillions of cells. Depriving it of that fuel source means it's not going to run as well or as long as it should. Your brain alone needs about 500 calories of carbs a day. It is the premium fuel for your brain to burn. Do you really want to make your brain run on a less than ideal fuel?

The first thing your body wants to do with carbs is burn them. Glucose (also given the unfortunate name of blood sugar) is used real-time by all of your cells. Glucose is most readily available when your body is actively digesting food. Between meals, if you fast or when you sleep, your body needs a backup battery to keep things running. That is where glycogen comes in. Your body will store about two pounds of glycogen (along with 4-6 pounds of water) in your liver and your muscles so you don't shut down when you're not eating.

Once your glycogen stores are full, your brown fat will burn carbs as body heat. The colder the temperature, the more energy your body has to expend keeping you warm. (We would still rather live in a warm climate.)

After those three things are addressed, then and only then will your body turn carbs into fat. This is not very energy efficient at all. It's much easier to store fat as fat than it is to convert carbs to fat.

In addition, going low-carb, which by definition means high-fat and high-protein, stresses the human system. Sure, you can lose weight in the short-term because you're cutting calories. But going low-carb is mortgaging your future health for short-term weight loss. It's not good for humans, no matter what fancy, fad-diet name is used. Of course, as a peak performer, you know better than to sacrifice your future for a small fleeting gain now.

What to do instead – Humans thrive on a diet that is about 80% whole-food starch (carbs). Fill your belly to your heart's content with real, recognizable foods: root veggies like sweet potatoes, grains like oats, whole wheat and quinoa, legumes (beans, peas, lentils), nuts and seeds. They will fill you up, keep you satisfied and keep your brain running like a champ. And you'll likely reach and maintain your ideal weight without ever feeling deprived.

*Not all carbs are created equal. We are talking here about whole-food plant carbs not loaded with butter or sour cream. All bets are off if you fill up on processed carbs that are loaded with sugar and fat and have no nutritional value like cakes, cookies and donuts. We don't want to hear, "I read a book that said carbs were good" as an excuse to eat half a birthday cake.

The bottom line – You can't trick the human body. Chemical flavors meant to mimic food aren't food and they are going to cause problems. Hunger is an ingrained survival instinct. Not eating whole-food carbs and using portion control is trying to tell 2.5 million years of human evolution to eat less. It is simply impossible to succeed by depriving yourself. Give your body the right amount of the correct fuel and it will hum along like that fine-tuned machine it is designed to be. It wants to be healthy. Stop fiddling with the gauges and let it!

How to Eat the Whole Food Muscle Way

How you eat is deeply ingrained in your subconscious mind. What you were fed as a child, when you were completely dependent on someone who you unquestionably trusted to give you what was best for you, is locked away as healthy and perfect. It most likely wasn't. As an adult you know that your mom, parent or caregiver was busy and overwhelmed and just doing their best to keep you alive and kinda happy. But that fact is lost on the part of your brain in charge of eating.

The foods of our childhood often have strong emotional components. My great-grandmother used to make a casserole with cheese, cream of mushroom (I think it was mushroom) soup and tater tots. As an adult I looked at the recipe and my logical brain thought "Why would anyone eat that? Yikes!" But deep in my emotional brain there are feelings of warmth, comfort, love and family associated with that casserole (I have very similar feelings for a family breakfast casserole). If my health and longevity didn't matter to me, or I wasn't aware of the health issues with eating it, or if I was addicted to short-term emotional gratification, I would make and eat those things without question.

Fortunately, I do know better. When those dishes are sitting on the buffet table at family gatherings, I can smile at the memories they bring up for me and not put any of it on my plate.

The first step

The first step to any journey to change is knowledge. If your conscious brain doesn't know that the foods you love and crave, emotionally or physically, are bad for you, why would you give them up? And even when you do know, sometimes the craving is just too much to bear (The challenges of the Pleasure Trap, emotional eating and Pavlovian eating discussed in the chapter **I Know I Should Eat Better, But...**)

The more you know, the better you will be at defending your desire to be healthy against your cravings (and your nagging family, friends and coworkers). But you know that or you wouldn't be reading this book. Let's assume you are at the point where you're ready to start making better choices for your health and longevity.

How do you eat now?

Are you an all-day grazer? Coffee first thing, something light and easy around 10 a.m., heavy lunch and dinner with snacking in the afternoon and late into the evening? Maybe you are a breakfast, snacking, appetizers, drinks, dinner person. You could be a whatever-is-easy and available person (This was me in my twenties. I would rather eat nothing than have to figure out food.). Does your eating pattern change on the weekends or depending on your schedule?

Every person we have ever coached has had an eating pattern. Some are messy and less than structured and others could tell us down to the minute when they ate what. Understanding your style is going to help you incorporate healthy choices. In our first consult meeting with a new client, we take notes about this so we can refer back to them. You might feel silly writing it down. But we suggest you do it anyway. Date it and keep it somewhere so you can refer back to it.

What our eating pattern looked like before and now

Before we moved to the Whole Food Muscle style of eating, we ate three meals a day plus snacks. We were doing something close to the Mediterranean diet (Not on purpose. We just tried to eat "clean.") and we tried to pay attention to portion control. It wasn't really working for us. We were both pretty fluffy, getting fluffier and our cholesterol was on the rise (My peak cholesterol reading was 256).

Now we eat a solid breakfast (see our oatmeal recipe) after our workout at 9:30 a.m. on weekdays, a nutrient-dense and large (read very filling) lunch around 2:30-ish and then something light in the evening if we feel like it. Russ is more likely to eat around dinner time than I am. When it's cold out, we are more likely to eat heavier, hot meals. In the summer, we are more active, but eat lighter and often raw (think huge salads). I have tracked my weight on a spreadsheet for clients to see and my monthly average weight drops a couple of pounds in the summer and then comes back up in the winter.

You might wonder what happened to our eating three solid meals a day. We have a couple of theories.

First – our bodies are getting WAY more nutrition than they used to, which means our cells aren't screaming for nutrients. **Second** – we are no longer fighting the inflammation and fatigue caused by our former way of eating, where we associated feeling tired and sluggish with hunger. And **third** – we have learned to recognize what actual hunger feels like.

We are not suggesting that we deprive ourselves or that we don't eat if we're hungry. Exactly the opposite. We DO eat when we're hungry. We just don't when we're not.

Don't be surprised if your eating pattern changes as you feed yourself more real food and become aware of your body's needs.

Make healthy food easy

If you don't have healthy food in the house, you can't eat it. If you have junk in the house, you will eat it. This is not news but it's amazing how often this reality is overlooked or ignored. Don't put temptation in your way. It makes it more likely you will fall victim to decision exhaustion, willpower fatigue, emotional eating and Pavlovian eating.

Donate, give away or toss the foods you no longer want to be eating and then don't buy them again. If you live in a home with someone who is unwilling to join you on this journey or is actively trying to sabotage you, this is going to be harder. And we don't want to hear the excuse, "But my kids..." Your kids don't need to be eating junk any more than you do. Feeding it to them is setting them up to have to retrain their taste buds as adults like you're doing now (We know that's some hard love. Truths are truths.).

Download the food staples list and the 24 snack ideas (*www.HowToFeedAHuman.com/downloads*) and fill your house with real food. It can be stuff that's easy to eat (you can microwave a sweet potato and put premade guacamole on it in five minutes) and ingredients for batch cooking something you can eat for a week

Join the Whole Food Muscle Club for meal ideas, cooking tips and recipes.

If you want to join our Whole Food Muscle Club and save over 50% off the regular member fee, go to *www.WholeFoodMuscle.com/bookdiscount* for the discount price as our thanks for buying this book.

Right about now your brain might be pushing back, "I don't have time for that!" We have said this before. We are going to say it again; if you outsource what you eat, you are trading time now for time being sick later and time in your coffin. As high performers we don't have to explain the flaw in that logic to you. Unless you have the money to hire a personal chef who understands this way of eating to cook for you, you need to take responsibility here. Step up to the plate and make it happen. There is no excuse for you to feed your body junk. It's that simple.

Pick a staple meal or two

When you have a meal or two that is your everyday go-to, you don't have to think about it. That's why we eat oatmeal with fruit and seeds every morning (we call it oatmeal, but there is more fruit, seeds and spices than oatmeal in it.). We know every day (except fasting days) when we get home from the gym, we are going to eat oatmeal. It's a foregone conclusion. On really rare occasions I will have something different. But Russ, never. He's eaten oatmeal for breakfast for 40 years. Why change now? We know we will be starting our day with an amazing load of nutrients and fiber that will keep us feeling full and focused for five-six hours (Longer for me. I would forget to eat lunch until early evening if Russ didn't text me to say, "Lunch?" from downstairs).

Your staple meal doesn't have to be oatmeal and it doesn't have to be breakfast. Maybe you like Buddha bowls. Maybe you like to eat a monster salad every day. Whatever works for you, always have those ingredients on hand and eat that thing without fail. It makes life easy and it's one less decision you have to make.

Caveat – Make sure you pick a staple meal that is high in nutrition and bulk. Choosing a low- nutrition, low-volume meal would be counterproductive.

Snack smart

There isn't really anything wrong with snacking per se. The idea of eating something light between meals just isn't a huge deal. But that's not how most people snack. Whole bags of potato chips, a complete box of cookies, two-thirds of a cake or a candy bar (or two or three) is hardly a "snack." If you are legitimately hungry, eat. Eat a snack or eat another meal. As long as it's real food, it's fine. The more nutrient-dense it is (nutrient-to-calorie ratio) the better. You can download our twenty-four healthy snack ideas list here: *www.HowToFeedAHuman.com/downloads*

The biggest takeaway about snacking is to make sure you legitimately know what hunger feels like.

> ***Don't be surprised if your eating pattern changes as you feed yourself more real food and become aware of your body's needs.***

Hunger versus toxic hunger

Dr. Joel Fuhrman coined the term "toxic hunger." He explains that the human body has two states: digesting food and not digesting food. When your body is digesting food, it is focused on doing just that. It takes about four hours for your body to digest an average meal. When it's not digesting food, it can focus on doing cleanup and repair. If you eat more often than every four hours or ingest a lot of animal protein, your body rarely gets out of the digestion phase, hardly having a chance to clean up toxins. Dr.

Fuhrman goes on to suggest that some of the symptoms that many of us associate with hunger, such as being "hangry," shaky or feeling nauseous are actually symptoms of your body trying to catch up on cleanup and repair. Unfortunately, as soon as we experience these types of symptoms, we eat, forcing our body to abandon cleanup and go back to digestion. This is one of the reasons intermittent fasting (discussed in detail in the **Intermittent Fasting FAQs** chapter) is thought to be good for us. It allows our body a chance to get caught up on toxic cleanup.

Add Whole-Plant Foods to What You're Currently Eating

When we first started moving towards the Whole Food Muscle Way, we never planned to be 100%. Our goal was to tweak our diet enough to lose the fluffy. But the more plants we ate, the better we felt and the more we learned, the more plants we wanted to eat. It took us six to eight months to end up being 100%. We started by putting chickpeas on our salads instead of chicken. We ate bean tacos instead of turkey. We made a point to eat our vegetables and starch (sweet potatoes and grains) first, before eating meat. This was the exact opposite of what both of us had been taught as athletes. We started splitting a chicken breast rather than each having one. We stopped buying eggs and milk. We made our oatmeal first with plant milk and then with water. Slowly animal products became the exception rather than the rule.

I kept a calendar and tracked how often I had meat, eggs or dairy (we weren't big processed food eaters, so that wasn't on the calendar) and color coded it to be able to see at a glance how many days a week I wasn't eating plants and to what extent. Eventually I stopped keeping the calendar because there weren't any animal products left to put on it.

We realized we were done with animal products the night we had friends over for dinner and made turkey tacos for them and bean tacos for ourselves.

At the end of the night, there was about a pound of turkey taco mixture leftover. We looked at each other and realized we weren't going to eat it. We tried to find someone to give it to, but it ended up in the trash. At that moment we realized, "If we won't eat it because it's unhealthy and we don't consider it food, what are we doing feeding it to our friends?" From then on, we started inviting our friends over to "eat plants." No one has ever said "no" or left hungry.

You could make similar small changes. Nothing says you have to go cold turkey (pun intended). Just start by incorporating the foods from our staples list (*www.HowToFeedAHuman.com/downloads*) into your diet. Eat them first. Over time you'll find they squeeze out the animal products. And you'll be surprised by how great you feel.

If you have a whole-plant food you already enjoy, add more of it to your diet.

One little word of caution – once you move to the Whole Food Muscle Way of eating, your taste buds and gut bacteria will change. The last time we ate nachos from our favorite place as a "treat," the cheese tasted like plastic. Our bodies have become so accustomed to not having to digest oil that we often get sick to our stomach when we eat vegan food at a restaurant. And we have had many clients report becoming physically ill after a cheat meal of meat or cheese.

Try meatless Monday or a few meatless meals

If you are currently eating meat, dairy or eggs three times (or more) a day, seven days a week, just making one day a week plant-based is going to introduce some great nutrition into your life. Pick one of the example meal plans in the **How We Eat** chapter or make up one of your own. Surely as a high-performance person, you can do one day a week.

It's pretty easy to switch your breakfast to the Whole Food Muscle Way. Just add oatmeal, seeds and fruit – magic! Choosing to put beans, lentils, nuts or seeds on your salad or in your pasta at lunch instead of chicken could make lunch meatless. Add in some of our Whole Food Muscle snacks (Go to *www.HowToFeedAHuman.com/downloads* to get your copy) and suddenly you're only eating one meat-meal a day. That is great progress!

If you can aim to eat about 80% plants, you'll be on a great track. Assuming you aren't using intermittent fasting (which we do recommend you look at doing), you are eating 21 meals a week, 80% would mean limiting your meat, dairy and egg consumption to four times a week. Some people choose to stay there. Others, like us, realize that's not optimal and find that they feel so good they want to eat more plants. As a high achiever, I'd be surprised if you ended up deciding to stay at 80% of anything.

Don't get hung up on what is "breakfast" food

If you have ever eaten cold pizza in the morning, you can't tell us that only certain foods are breakfast foods. If you want to eat sweet potato lasagna for breakfast, do so. If oatmeal for dinner will hit the spot – no worries! There is no reason to eat certain nutrients at specific times. Your body is happy to have them whenever and in whatever order you send them.

Interestingly, before we made the switch to eating the Whole Food Muscle Way, Russ wouldn't be able to sleep if he ate something heavy before bed. He would be bloated and miserable. Now that we are eating 100% plants, he has had times where he has eaten a lot of bulk and felt very full, but he doesn't feel uncomfortably bloated. Sometimes he will lose five pounds between going to bed and getting up in the morning! We share that to say, you may not have to worry about how late you eat unless you are incorporating intermittent fasting into your lifestyle.

Try new foods

We have seen numbers varying between 20,000 and 80,000 for types of plants on our planet that are edible by humans. We are pretty sure there are a least a few you haven't tried. When we tell people we eat only plants, they often ask incredulously (right after "where do you get your protein?"), "What DO you eat?" The variety in our diet has increased dramatically since we made the switch because we try new recipes and add new spices. That's not to say we have loved everything we tried. But we have found many new things we do like and the process of trying them is fun.

We did a survey asking what foods our clients eat now that they had either never heard of or never tried before they started moving towards the Whole Food Muscle Way. You can see their responses by downloading new foods to try here: *www.HowToFeedAHuman.com/downloads*. Perhaps make it a goal to try something new from this list once a week for a while.

Don't be shy about buying a new ingredient. You could even be really brave and sign up to have a subscription box of ugly veggies sent to you (We have had to use Google to figure out what something was and how to eat it.). You never know what you're going to get and you just might find a new favorite.

Don't try to fool yourself

There is nothing more disappointing than making a "cheese" sauce from potatoes and carrots that looked SO good in the video and then realizing it tastes nothing like cheese. You aren't going to be able to fool your taste buds without a lot of heavy and unhealthy oils. Faux meats, cheeses and spreads, although vegan, are not healthy. You want to eat whole foods, not processed food-stuff that happens to be made from plants but is supposed to taste like animals. That is one of the challenges of eating at vegan restaurants. Your health is not their focus. Faux foods are fine if they help you transition or if you're in a pinch while eating out. But you will likely find they make you feel poorly because of the amount of oil in them.

There are plenty of whole-plant based dishes that you will love. Even Russ' mom loves it when we bring food to her house. She has said many times, "I can't believe how flavorful the food you eat is. I always thought it would be bland." Give your taste buds a week or so to unclog from the sludge that is the Standard American Diet and you'll be amazed at the burst of flavors real food can create in your mouth.

Engage with people on the same journey

Everything is easier when you surround yourself with like-minded people. While the journey to better productivity, health and longevity is gaining popularity, there are still a lot of places where you might feel you're on an island by yourself. Join groups and communities with other plant-based people.

We offer several options as part of the Whole Food Muscle Club. Ask questions, share your successes, challenges and suggestions, and even chat with other Whole Food Muscle members. If you want to join our Whole Food Muscle Club and save over 50% off the regular member fee, go to *www.WholeFoodMuscle.com/bookdiscount* for the discount price as our thanks for buying this book.

Having a place you know you can ask questions without being attacked, or expected to already know everything is key. Be aware that vegan groups are NOT that place. And many public groups calling themselves plant-based or vegan are not user-friendly. Don't allow fanatics and better-than-you folks to sabotage your journey. Our groups are monitored. Trolls, meanies and know-it-alls are not tolerated.

Know enough to be able to defend your choice with science

You are going to get pushback; that is just a given. People who don't understand and don't want to understand are going to question what you are doing and why. As soon as you mention anything about eating only plants, suddenly everyone you know will act like they have three PhDs in nutrition and human biochemistry. They will NEED to tell you why what you're doing is a horrible idea and that you won't get enough protein (they have no idea what they are talking about). In extreme cases they may call you names and be actively obnoxious. We have heard and experienced some horror stories. You have two choices, used individually or in combination, don't care and walk away or have responses ready for a few of the most popular oppositions people will throw at you.

Here are a few and how we answer them:

- **Being vegan isn't healthy.** You're right. Being a junk-food vegan is most certainly not healthy. I am not vegan which is an ethical stance that includes not eating animals. I eat the Whole Food Muscle Way. Health and longevity studies show it to be the optimal way of eating for humans. There is a TED talk about the Blue Zones that's a good summary. Then give them a copy of this book.

- **Everyone has to die at some point.** True. Not everyone has to live the last 20 years of their lives being kept half alive by Big Pharma. I'd like to live healthy and vibrant for as long as possible.

- **I know so-and-so who ate red meat, smoked and drank every day and lived to be 95.** That is called survivor's bias. I know lots of people who ride motorcycles without helmets and are alive. That doesn't make it a smart choice.

- **Where will you get your protein?** The human body doesn't need nearly as much protein as people think. 10% of calories is plenty. Eating the Whole Food Muscle Way, I get that and more. Plus, humans are very good at recycling their own amino acids as they wear out and need to be replaced. There is no such thing as a protein-deficiency ward in hospitals. As long as I'm ingesting enough calories, I will get enough protein. If you want to be snarky, you can then ask them where they get their fiber. But that can lead to a whole conversation about bathroom habits so...

- **Carbs will make you fat.** The foods you think of as "carbs"– processed cakes, cookies and donuts contain more fat than carbs and the carbs in them have had all the nutrients removed to make them shelf-stable. The few whole-food carbs most people eat are buried under a mountain of animal fat (think, loaded baked potato – don't blame the potato for making you fluffy when it's the loaded you put on it.). That's not what I'm eating. Whole-food carbs attached to their fiber as nature intended are a great fuel source are loaded with nutrients and keep me feeling full. They aren't going to be turned into fat by my body.

- **I could never eat like a rabbit.** I don't either. Rabbits don't eat starch.

- **You have to live a little.** "Dyin' ain't much of a livin'." (Hat tip to Clint Eastwood in the movie, Outlaw Josey Wales)

- **I would always be hungry.** If you were, you wouldn't be eating enough. That's the beauty of eating this way. High-nutrient density and low-calorie density means you always get to eat until you're full.

- **The Inuit lived on whale blubber.** "Lived" yes. Thrived? Not hardly. They die before they are sixty and have the heart disease you would

> expect from eating a diet high in animal fat. You might also find it interesting that they don't live in ketosis. They get enough carbs to teeter on the edge of survival from the glycogen in the muscle they eat. By contrast, people living in the Blue Zones where humans live the longest, many over 100, eat mostly whole-plant foods and are thriving.

There you have it. That's all the building blocks you need to start feeding yourself like the high-performance human you are and deal with the stones and arrows people will try to sling at you. All you have to add is the desire to be at the top of your game, which we know you already have.

The more plants we ate, the better we felt and the more we learned, the more plants we wanted to eat.

I Know I Should Eat Better, But...

As a high performer you know that any achievement requires intention and focus. You've likely used that strategy many times in your life. But when it comes to your health, somehow all of that determination and drive gets lost. Maybe you even have a strategy to improve your health but you're failing at the execution. There are several excuses and psychological hurdles that can get in the way and knowing what they are will help you overcome them.

No time/too busy

This is one of the most popular excuses for not doing just about everything. But, as a high performer, what could possibly be SO important in your life that your health is worth giving away for it? We all know the answer to that – nothing. Nothing in your life is important enough to give your health away.

We have to get over the mindset that feeding ourselves is an inconvenience (a story made up and pushed on us by the food industry). Moving past that barrier is pretty straightforward once you understand the lies we've been told by those trying to profit from what we eat.

How much more time does it take to eat well anyway? Inhaling fast "food" isn't actually eating. Being a high achiever means allotting time for things that matter and prioritizing. Put your health at the top of the list. No excuses.

The addiction to distraction

With the ability to pull entertainment out of our pocket at any moment, few of us spend any time allowing our brain to just wander. It is thought of as a waste of time. But you know that's not true. You've likely read and heard about the benefits of meditation. I'm not going to suggest you start meditating (that's in plenty of other books). But I am going to suggest your feeling that you are too overwhelmed to spend even a moment thinking about what you are eating could be caused by the never-ending stream of incoming information into your brain. Radio, TV, computer, phone, work meetings, books, papers and social media are all a constant barrage of incoming information.

And your brain gets addicted to it and wants more. If you're like most people, you have information coming in right up until you fall asleep and it starts again the moment you wake up. Do you eat while scrolling through your phone or on your computer? The answer is very likely "yes." How do you expect to be able to hear your body tell you you're full? You can't. You'll just eat until your plate is empty. And if it's loaded with standard fare, you'll have eaten entirely too much fat, sugar and salt, and not nearly enough nutrients.

What if you curbed your addiction to distraction and took a moment to think about eating? Are you actually hungry? How hungry? But hungry for what? Is what you are about to eat nutritious fuel that will give you the energy you need AND increase your health and longevity? Or is it just junk to stuff in your mouth without thinking?

If you don't stop to think about it there is no way you can make a choice, you're too distracted.

Eating by least resistance/on autopilot

How often do you eat the same junk-food thing or at the unhealthy same place because you don't have to think about it? Do you walk the same path through the grocery store, picking up the same things without any real thought? Why is something tied directly to your health being handled so dismissively? Perhaps a little more focus is in order. You could decide to make healthy choices by rote, like we eat oatmeal every morning.

Decision exhaustion

You likely know that some of the most successful people in the world make an effort to limit the number of decisions they have to make every day. Some even go so far as wearing the same thing on a daily basis just to avoid thinking about clothing choices. Studies suggest each one of us makes upwards of 30,000 decisions a day. Assuming you sleep at least six hours, that means you are making 28 decisions a minute! How is that even possible? While it seems unlikely, a Cornell study found we make about 225 decisions a day about food alone. Talk about exhausting!

When your brain gets tired of making decisions, you're going to fall back on what is easy, quick and convenient and doesn't require any thought. This could be one of the reasons your healthy eating plan is always going to start on Monday, but never actually starts.

Willpower fatigue

Most diets rely on willpower to keep you from eating things you shouldn't. But over time, your willpower becomes exhausted. If you've ever done a great job of eating healthy during the day, but then binged on anything and everything you could find once the sun set, you have been a victim of willpower fatigue. You can't really bolster your willpower to make it last longer. But you can put systems and knowledge in place that will allow you to make food choices based on something other than your ability to resist unhealthy, tempting foods. That's why you're reading this book.

Chasing short-term pleasure/gratification

Humans have evolved with a procreate-today-because-you-may-die-tomorrow mentality. That's great for survival of the species, but not so great for the long-term health and survival of you as an individual. This outlook rears its head in the dopamine (pleasure chemical in our brain) we get from eating fatty, sweet, salty foods. It is also what makes us feel deprived when we try to use our willpower to not eat those things.

Humans have evolved with a procreate-today-because-you-may-die-tomorrow mentality. That's great for survival of the species, but not so great for the long-term health and survival of you as an individual.

And food companies know it! They have spent billions of dollars figuring out how they can purposefully tap into our pleasure center by manipulating "food" to make us crave it, unable to stop eating it once we start and miss it when we don't have it. Great for their profits. Horrible for our health.

Emotional eating

Negative emotions like sadness, stress, unhappiness and anxiety aren't fun. Since eating releases pleasure chemicals in our brains, it's easy to drown our sorrows under fat, sugar and salt. Eating ice cream and drinking alcohol is considered so normal after a break up, there are memes about it. For most people, it is easier to bury difficult emotions than it is to feel them and deal with them.

But what is really curious is we also eat when we are happy. Celebrations and holidays are associated with food: birthday cakes, fancy dinners and wedding receptions. When was the last time you got together with anyone and there wasn't food involved? Any and all emotion, good, bad or indifferent is a reason to put food, most likely processed sugar and fat, into our bodies.

Pavlovian eating/by habit

You know about Pavlov and his dogs that would salivate at the sound of a bell. But did you know that same response is making you eat foods you know are bad for you when you're not hungry?

Consider this:

You've been busy working. You look up and it's 1:45. Suddenly you're starving. Why? You weren't hungry five minutes ago.

You're at the movies or watching your favorite TV show. What are you eating? Why? You likely aren't actually hungry.

You're at a social event. There's a buffet of finger "food." You stand while talking and munching. Why? Are you hungry? Is that really food? Most likely not.

Habit. That's why. We've trained our brains to eat even when we aren't hungry. We eat when the clock says to, not when our stomach does. We eat in front of the TV or at the movies because that's just what we do. We eat in social settings because that's the norm.

Do you even remember what it feels like to actually be hungry? To eat when your body says you should and to stop when you've had enough? In all likelihood the answer is "no."

The world is full of triggers that make us eat unconsciously. But you are smarter than a dog. In fact, you're likely smarter than most humans. Put an end to Pavlovian eating. Your gut and your butt will thank you!

Fear of missing out

You're out with friends or business colleagues and someone orders several plates of appetizers for the table. You watch as everyone around you has their fingers covered in chicken wing sauce. They eat fried cheese, fried spring rolls, fried shrimp and whatever other fried things are on the table. (Why are appetizers ALWAYS fried?) They are all talking animatedly and look like they are having a great time. You want that too. And somehow your unconscious brain associates the good time they are having with the unhealthy things they are eating. It smells good. Your caveman brain says it is calorie dense, so great for survival.

A few hours later you're on your way home and your gut hurts. You knew you shouldn't have eaten that stuff. You even told yourself you weren't going to. But you did. And now you're miserable. The fear-of-missing-out virus got you.

Peer pressure

You might think at this point in your life peer pressure is a thing of the past or at the very least you would be immune to it. But, sadly, that is not the case. These are a few things we have heard from grown adults:

- You always eat so healthy. This one time won't matter.
- You have to live a little.
- You make me feel bad about myself when you eat so healthy.
- I know so-and-so who is 92 years old and has eaten junk, smoked and drank his/her whole life.
- There will be a study next week that says bacon is good for you.
- You're skinny. I'm jealous that you can eat whatever you want.
- I know you don't usually eat this, but I made it and you HAVE to try it.
- Don't be awkward and cause a scene. Just eat normal food for once.
- But it's your birthday/Thanksgiving/Christmas/insert excuse here.
- You act like you're better than the rest of us.
- You're too thin! You should eat.
- You really can't afford to lose any more weight.

All of those comments represent someone directly trying to get you to do something you don't want to. Some of them are embarrassing. Some are rude. All are thoughtless. Have a plan for how you want to handle such things. Sometimes just laughing and shaking your head is enough. Sometimes having a good comeback is in order. And sometimes you may have to call the person out, either publicly, "Really? Peer pressure?" or "Are you purposefully trying to embarrass me?" or by pulling them aside and having a private conversation.

Feeling deprived

"I don't feel well. I don't sleep well. And I have celiac disease. I DESERVE to eat whatever I want," a client who was easily 60 pounds overweight stated staunchly. He felt like he was deprived in so many areas of his life that food was his one joy. But it was killing him (hence his not feeling or sleeping well).

Reading the above, you likely had one of two responses. You either empathize with him or you think he's acting like a petulant child. Feeling like we "deserve" to eat whatever we want and that there shouldn't be any consequences leads to unhappiness. When your mind thinks, "I can't have that" there is an immediate feeling of being robbed of something that should be ours and our inner petulant child stomps their foot in frustration.

Instead of thinking, "I can't," it is more productive to think, "I choose not to." Choosing allows your inner child to feel in control and your successful, grownup self can smile knowingly because you have the knowledge WHY you choose not to.

The Pleasure Trap

Dr. Douglas Lisle, Director of Research for the TrueNorth Health Center, developed the idea (described in his book, The Pleasure Trap) that we are trapped by the way our brains interpret and become normalized to pleasure. The first bite you eat of something really good brings a large spike in pleasure chemicals in your brain. But as you keep eating it, your enjoyment levels off and then dips back to baseline. To get that same high you will need something different or better. Humans have the same response to using drugs. That is true when you eat a dessert and true across the spectrum of foods you eat.

As a teenager, many of us start to get more freedom in our food choices. And most of us make some pretty awful choices. At the beginning, it is exciting and new. But then those choices become normal. When we get into our early twenties, beer, pizza, subs and fast food are so normal that we don't even think about it. They are not providing the same level of food high. They don't bring pleasure. They are just what we eat. Our taste buds and our brain have acclimated to the fat, sugar and salt. And real, healthy, nutritious food now seems bland and boring.

To get back to eating what your body actually needs, you'll have to wean yourself off of the junk food. And it's then that you realize just how addicted you really are.

When your mind thinks, "I can't have that" there is an immediate feeling of being robbed of something that should be ours and our inner petulant child stomps their foot in frustration.

Self-discipline

You are a high-performance person. Everything in your life is done with precision and purpose. You might even be the type of person who wastes time on a specific schedule. But how you nourish your body is not under control. It's too easy to grab the pizza provided during the lunch meeting or order the chicken Alfredo, telling yourself the fib that it's healthy because it's chicken. All of the other excuses and hurdles meld together and overwhelm your self-discipline when it comes to food.

Like any area of your life, you can improve your ability to make better choices by understanding what is holding you back, gaining the knowledge you need, creating a plan to do something different and overcoming the obstacles to your successful execution of that plan. Action and implementation. You do it in other areas of your life. Your health and longevity shouldn't be any different.

Intermittent Fasting FAQs

Intermittent fasting, sometimes abbreviated IF and also called "time-restricted eating" has been gaining in popularity in recent years. It is used both as a method of dieting and to improve health and longevity. When we started researching health and longevity nutrition, we were introduced to intermittent fasting by a doctor. After looking into the science of it, we decided it was right for us (more on how we implemented it at the end of this chapter) and many of our clients use it as part of eating the Whole Food Muscle Way. There are several ways to implement it in your life if you believe it is the right choice for you.

What is intermittent fasting?

Intermittent fasting is the conscious decision to eat at certain times and not eat at others. Basically, it is patterned eating, the opposite of grazing. Drinking water is a MUST! We will explain the details of different styles of intermittent fasting below. But it is important to realize that fasting does not give you the freedom to eat whatever you want with abandon when you do eat. Nutrition and food quality are still the heavy-hitters of human health and longevity.

The history of intermittent fasting

Fasting has been part of the human condition since the beginning of time. This is mostly because food just wasn't always available. Humans, like other animals, ate when they could find food and didn't when they couldn't. In recent centuries, fasting became part of many religions, but other than that, it has fallen by the wayside as food became available on every street corner in the Western world. However, the constant access to ever cheaper, but less nourishing, calories has come at a health price. We are fatter and sicker than ever. The more we diet, the fatter we end up and rates of metabolic diseases like diabetes, heart disease, obesity, high blood pressure and high cholesterol are skyrocketing. Our bodies could really use a break from the nearly nonstop processing of food.

Why intermittent fasting is good for you

When our bodies are processing food, the pancreas releases insulin to move glucose (blood sugar) from the blood into the cells where it can be used as energy. When there is insulin in the system, your body is not burning fat because there is plenty of fuel in the form of glucose. When you fast, all of your glucose gets used up and your body shifts to using glycogen (stored in the liver and muscle cells) for fuel and your insulin levels begin to drop. After six to eight hours you run out of glycogen and your body must start burning fat (Don't worry. That's how it's designed to work).

Not having insulin in the system and burning fat helps with insulin sensitivity. It also gives your body a chance to clean up cells that aren't functioning at their peak level, called "zombie" cells (yes, really). They are there, but they aren't doing their job. When your body isn't focused on processing food, it gets a chance to notice, "Hmm, this cell is not in good shape" or "This one didn't replicate correctly" and it can dispose of them. Just like your computer can only run a defrag to clean up the memory when you're not working on it.

Plus, the calorie restriction that happens naturally with intermittent fasting and the resulting ideal body weight has been shown to increase longevity.

Will intermittent fasting help with weight loss?

Yes. Intermittent Fasting has been demonstrated to be as useful in creating weight loss as calorie restriction diets and many people find it to be much easier. We have had clients report that it takes less willpower to say, "not yet" for a scheduled period of time than it does to say, "just a little" all of the time (not to mention that portion-control diets lower metabolism). We have a client who has lost 80+ pounds using a version of 16/8 intermittent fasting (explained below) and eating mostly the Whole Food Muscle Way.

The upside of intermittent fasting as compared to calorie restriction is that the fat-to-muscle ratio being lost is better. Typically, 25% of weight lost is muscle. However, with intermittent fasting that drops to 10%.

Will intermittent fasting make me too thin?

For those who struggle to eat enough to maintain a healthy weight, either due to an eating disorder or just not being big eaters, intermittent fasting is likely not an ideal choice. However, for the rest of us, using intermittent fasting does not seem to cause our bodies to get too thin. It took us about six months of intermittent fasting while moving towards the Whole Food Muscle Way for us to reach our ideal weight. Since then, our weight has been stable within a few pounds. With our active lifestyle, it could be assumed that if intermittent fasting was going to make someone too thin, it would be us. But that has not been the case at all.

What we have noticed is we are both leaner in a way we never were before. We have more muscle definition than we did at a similar weight when we were younger and not fasting or eating this way. We both have our abs back, which has been a nice surprise.

Will I binge eat when I break my fast?

It is unlikely that you will binge eat when you break your fast, assuming that you choose good quality, nutritious foods. If you eat highly processed foods loaded with fat, it's going to be REALLY easy to eat to the point that you are miserable and take in WAY more calories than you need. However, studies indicate that most people ingest about 10% more calories after a fast than they normally would. Which means that you're 90% down from what your normal intake would have been had you not fasted.

Will intermittent fasting ruin my metabolism?

No. Your metabolism does not respond to fasting the same way it does to calorie restriction. In calorie restriction there is a reduced amount of fuel available over a long period of time. During that time your body learns, "There is consistently only this amount of fuel available. We had better conserve our energy" and turns down your metabolism. This can lead to the frustrating experience of a weight loss plateau, followed by gaining weight, even though calorie intake is still low.

By contrast, intermittent fasting teaches your body that there are always plenty of calories available on average. They just aren't available ALL the time. So, your metabolism keeps humming right along, doing what your body is designed to do – burn fat when fasting (That's how you stay alive through the night). In fact, your metabolism may go up a bit while fasting because your body thinks, "Hey! Get off your backside and go find some food!"

Will intermittent fasting lead to an eating disorder?

No. An eating disorder is an emotional or psychological condition that manifests in the way a person engages with food. Intermittent fasting will not CAUSE someone who does not have an eating disorder to suddenly have one. However, if someone has an eating disorder, intermittent fasting could be used as an excuse to engage in disordered eating.

I have a history of disordered eating, having had anorexic tendencies in my early to mid-twenties. When I decided to add intermittent fasting, I was careful to pay attention to my thoughts about food, eating and my body. Fortunately, my emotional anxiety due to lack of control and having no say in my life in my twenties has been resolved. I have not experienced any desire, thoughts or internal pressure to engage in disordered eating in almost two decades. Intermittent fasting has not changed that (it has however helped bring back the body I remembered and love).

If you engage or have engaged in disordered eating, please work with a professional to address the underlying factors prior to adding intermittent fasting to your lifestyle. Discuss any unhealthy thoughts about eating, not eating and your body that come up for you with them.

Fasting does not give you the freedom to eat whatever you want with abandon when you do eat.

How intermittent fasting helps diabetes

Because intermittent fasting gives your body a break from insulin and reduces fat in the system, it helps with insulin sensitivity. It also helps with diabetes as a mechanism of weight loss. Dr. McDougall talks about patients on the verge of amputation showing up at his program in wheelchairs and walking out after using a ten- to thirty-day water fast and then following a healthy plant-based diet. Clearly, fasting of this nature should only be done under the strict supervision of a doctor knowledgeable in both fasting and diabetes.

If you are taking diabetic medications, work closely with your doctor to monitor your medication needs. Adding fasting and / or moving toward the Whole Food Muscle Way can rapidly reduce your medication needs.

Because intermittent fasting gives your body a break from insulin and reduces fat in the system, it helps with insulin sensitivity. It also helps with diabetes as a mechanism of weight loss.

Can I work out while intermittent fasting?

Absolutely. When you first start fasting you might find that your body is a little cranky about working out, particularly if you typically eat before you work out. That is just your body being in the habit of not having to burn fat. Start out by doing one of your less strenuous workouts on a fasting day. We work out five days a week, regardless of it being a fasting day or not. It took a few weeks for our bodies to adapt, but now we don't even think about it. I have done hard cardio on fasting days and Russ has done legs (his most strenuous workout – not that all his workouts aren't strenuous!) without a problem. Of course, make sure you stay hydrated while working out. That's good advice whether you're fasting or not.

What breaks an intermittent fast?

Anything that causes metabolic activity in your body breaks your fast. That means anything with calories or anything your body thinks SHOULD have calories. Chemicals that make your brain think it's getting calories (i.e., artificial sweeteners) have been shown to turn the system on. You're going to want to avoid both fake and real calories. Most experts agree that plain tea, water and unflavored sparkling water are fine. There is some disagreement about black coffee, but generally most seem to think it is fine to drink while fasting. However, be aware that the acid on an empty stomach might not be the best option.

Can I chew gum while intermittent fasting?

Because of the artificial sweeteners in gum, we do not recommend chewing gum while fasting (see the above paragraph).

When should I eat after intermittent fasting?

When you eat depends on what style of fasting you choose and what works best for your lifestyle. There really is no wrong way to add intermittent fasting to your life.

What should I eat after intermittent fasting?

The best choice for breaking a fast is something rich in nutrients. If you are eating the Whole Food Muscle Way, that isn't going to be a problem. If you are still eating animal products, you will want to stay away from them to break your fast. They are going to sit heavy in your gut and, because you are hungry, it will be SUPER easy to eat way too much.

We laugh at ourselves because when we break our fast, we want to eat all the things! Everything in the house looks and tastes amazing (a side benefit of fasting is your taste buds go on high alert and everything is yummier)! Inevitably, I end up having to put some of what I make back in the fridge because my eyes are bigger than my stomach after fasting.

Which intermittent fast works best?

The short answer is whichever style you can make work with your life on a consistent basis. There are benefits to fasting for as little as 12 hours and they go up as you hit 18 hours, 24 hours and 36 hours (for the record, we have NEVER fasted 36 hours straight). Fat burning tends to be at its peak between 16 and 24 hours into a fast and there have been some studies that suggest that 24-hour fasts are best for weight loss. But that certainly does not mean that shorter fasts aren't beneficial.

Is a juice fast the same as intermittent fasting?

No. A juice "fast" is no different for your body's metabolic level than eating because there are calories to process. In fact, it's not as good for you as eating whole-food. Juicing is not part of the Whole Food Muscle Way of eating. Details about why can be found in the **Juicing is NOT the Answer** chapter.

Intermittent fasting – where to start

You are already fasting. Every night when you go to sleep your body burns through your glucose stores and into your glycogen. Depending on how long you go between eating at night and eating in the morning, you might even start burning fat. If you want to start consciously using intermittent fasting, you just have to stretch that time window out a bit.

It is possible that you could just skip breakfast and you'd have a 16-or-so hour fast.

There are a few different styles of intermittent fasting. None is really better than another. Remember to drink plenty of water to stay well hydrated while fasting.

- 16/8 or using a feeding window. This is likely the easiest way to ease into intermittent fasting because you can just skip breakfast every day. It is called 16/8 because you fast sixteen hours a day and feed during an eight-hour window. Example: you would eat all of your meals between noon and 8 p.m. Some people push that even farther. We have a client who eats only one meal a day between 4 p.m. and 8 p.m. pretty much every day. She has been doing it for a little more than a year at this point and last we heard she was down 80 pounds. She is also mostly eating the Whole Food Muscle Way.

- 5-2. This method of fasting was made popular by the BBC documentary, Eat, Fast and Live Longer (available on YouTube, except in the UK). With this method you eat normally five days a week and fast on two non-consecutive days. On your fasting days you are allowed 500-600 calories. Some suggest eating all of your calories at once. Others say it's okay to split them up.

  This is the style of fasting we started with and we ate all of our calories at one time. Our logic being if the goal is to eliminate insulin, why would you eat 250 calories in the middle of your fast?

- Alternate-day fasting. Just like it sounds, you eat every other day. But that means you're fasting three or four whole days every week. That seems like a lot to us.

- 24-hour fasts. You fast for one or two periods of 24 hours weekly. We aren't sure when it happened, we didn't ever talk about it, but this is the style of fasting we do now. Somewhere along the way we moved from eating 500 calories on a fasting day, to fasting for about 24 hours and then eating a regular meal.

- Multi-day water fasts. Instead of fasting on a weekly basis you could do three consecutive days every month. That doesn't sound even a little bit fun to us (I would be intolerably cranky). For very ill patients, long (30+ days) water fasts have shown positive benefits. HOWEVER (this is really important), we DO NOT recommend fasting for more than about 36 hours without the supervision of a doctor who has specific knowledge about fasting.

What is the downside to intermittent fasting?

Most experts agree that there really is no health downside to intermittent fasting. People fast all the time before procedures and getting blood work done. Doing it regularly just extends the benefits. The only real negative is being cranky if you are fasting more than about twelve hours. Once your body figures out how fasting works and learns to burn fat without complaining about it, that crankiness goes away. It gets somewhat better after the first week but it might take up to six weeks to be really gone.

If you're worried that you'll get hungry and that the hunger feeling will build until you're ready to eat your arm (or your neighbor's arm), don't worry. That's not how hunger works. Sure, your stomach might growl at you (we have found that bubbly water helps with that) and you might think, "I'm hungry." But drink some water, work on a project or get engaged in something you enjoy and hunger will take a break. Eventually it will be more of, "Hey, we could eat" and you'll think, "Yeah, I know. We'll do that later."

Intermittent fasting – The Whole Food Muscle Way

When we started fasting, we chose the 5-2 method and decided that Wednesdays and Saturdays would be our fasting days. It only took us about two weeks to realize that fasting on a Saturday was really bad for our social life. Fortunately, we have a couple of bike riding friends — shout out to Jim and Steph — who put up with us biking with them and then hanging out at their house to visit and just drinking water rather than having lunch like we usually did. So, we switched our days to Mondays and Thursdays. That has worked well for us.

A side benefit of fasting is your taste buds go on high alert and everything is yummier!

We have tried having our fasting day meal as breakfast (about 9:30 a.m.) and as an early dinner (about 4 p.m.). We have found that 4 p.m. works better for us. This is mostly because I don't like going to bed hungry.

When we were doing the "real" 5-2, a 500-600 calorie meal might be a sweet potato with hummus or oatmeal with fruit (no seeds). Now that we are doing 24 hours two days a week (still Mondays and Thursdays), we typically fast between 22 and 26 hours depending on when we stop eating the night before and what time we break our fast and eat a regular meal. Often we eat whatever I batch cooked the weekend before, plus a salad of some kind.

Interestingly, we noticed just recently that in addition to our regular 24-hour fasts, it is common for us to eat dinner around 6:00 at night and then not eat again until breakfast at 9:30 a.m. Which means we are also doing a 15.5/8.5 type fast on a pretty regular basis. We have also observed we aren't nearly as hungry as we used to be when we were eating a more Mediterranean-style diet. We think that is because we are getting FAR more nutrients than we used to and our cells are happy. Of course, we are also both at our ideal weight now, so we don't have to feed the extra pounds of chunky-monkey we were carrying around.

We have found intermittent fasting to be a positive in our lives and we highly encourage it as part of the Whole Food Muscle Way. Give it a try. You might be surprised how easy it is and how good you feel.

The Psychology of Eating – Getting Your Brain to Agree

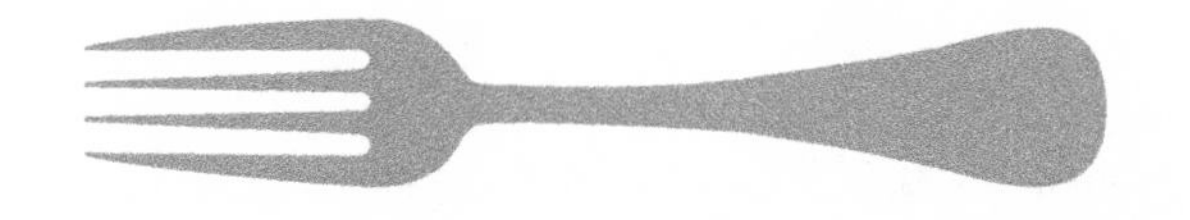

Portion Control Shouldn't be a Thing

"Eat less." "Control your portion size." "Calories in, calories out." "Use a smaller plate." "Eat more slowly." "Chew each bite 100 times." "Eat in moderation."

The amount of advice we see on how to trick the human body into not gaining and holding onto fat makes us want to bang our heads in frustration. Portion control is telling 2.5 million years of human evolution to eat less. It's not going to work. Humans are DESIGNED to average out to eating exactly how much we need – no more, no less. But there is a HUGE piece of the puzzle that has been removed from the game; we no longer eat the food we are designed to eat. Instead we are eating designer food that takes zero effort to obtain. That's a problem and it rigs the game against us.

The good news is, once you understand how the human body works, you don't have to try to trick it. You can just eat until you've had enough.

Here's why portion control doesn't work:

Your body can't count calories. A calorie is the amount of energy required to raise the temperature of a gram of water one degree Celsius. Shockingly the human body has no way to figure that out. When your logical brain counts calories, the rest of the human system laughs.

Your stretch receptors will not be denied. Your stomach feels full when the stretch receptors say you've put enough in there. It's about volume (made up by fiber). The calorie density doesn't matter that much to your stomach.

We are designed to eat food that needs to be chewed. One thing we've noticed since moving toward eating this way is that it takes longer to eat – and that's a GOOD thing! Plant foods have fiber in them that requires chewing. Chewing activates the saliva glands, which is the first step in healthy digestion, and gives the stretch receptors time to adjust to the food coming in. There is no reason to "wait 20 minutes and see if you're still hungry" when you eat food that actually has to be chewed.

Cells need nutrition. Nothing else matters. There are A LOT of edible products out there that have zero nutritional value. You can eat all the junk you want and your body is going to say, "I'm still hungry." When we talk about eating only plants, people often ask, "Where do you get your protein?" That's not even a concern, all plants have protein (more on that in **The Protein Cult** chapter). The big concern if you aren't eating plants is, "Where are you getting your nutrients?"

Portion control is telling 2.5 million years of human evolution to eat less. It's not going to work.

Most people do portion control by not eating veggies and starch. It never ceases to amaze us how often people will eat an entire chicken breast, hunk of steak or fish fillet and leave the broccoli and potato on their plate in the name of "portion control." Full disclosure: we used to do the same thing before we knew better. That is exactly backwards. Eat the veggie and the starch. In fact, eat two servings. Then decide if you really NEED the fat and cholesterol in the animal product.

Most people have no idea what it feels like to be hungry. Hunger is mostly a thing of the past in the Western world. We eat because "it's time." We eat because food is available. We eat mindlessly. We eat socially. We eat emotionally. We eat junk. We eat fast. We eat unhealthily. And it's killing us.

Forget portion control. Figure out what it feels like to be hungry, feed your body nutritious food it can actually use to build healthy cells. Don't give it junk food, animal fat and cholesterol it has to fight to process.

- Pick anything from some or all of these food groups and dig in!
- Legumes (beans and peas)
- Leaves (lettuce and spinach)
- Bulbs (onions and garlic)
- Flowers (broccoli and cauliflower)
- Whole grains (kamut, barley and oats)
- Roots (beets and potatoes)
- Stems (celery and asparagus)
- Nuts/seeds (walnuts, pumpkin seeds. Interestingly, quinoa is also a seed)
- Mushrooms and spices.

Eat until you've had enough and then stop. Easy.

Why Moderation Doesn't Work

Humans have an incredible power to see only what they want to see and deny any information to the contrary. If all else fails, justify, justify, justify. We see it A LOT when talking to people about their desire to live a long, healthy life versus their desire to eat, drink and be merry Somehow there is a disconnect between eating healthy and being merry. We and many people we know are both.

One of the most common justifications we hear when someone admits the choices they make aren't the healthiest of options:

"Well, everything in moderation, right?" followed by a shrug or a chuckle.

No. Not everything in moderation. That is ridiculous.

The problem with moderation is it doesn't actually mean anything. Where is the line between moderation and excess? How would you know if you crossed it? How far do you have to go to realize you have exceeded it? What are the short-term and long-term consequences of breaching the mark? What if, by the time you realized you had overdone it, it was too late to reverse the damage?

> ***The problem with moderation is it doesn't actually mean anything.***

There are no answers to those questions because the definition of moderation is "without excess." Whether something is in excess or not depends on personal opinion. It's like the line between hot and cold. There are no hard and fast rules.

- When someone says they want to continue doing something in moderation we hear:
- "I'm happy hitting myself with this hammer."
- "I want to continue this habit even though I know it's bad for me."
- "I'm not as unhealthy as other people."
- "I'm okay with this level of unhealthy in my life."
- "The amount I do this harmful thing isn't a big deal."
- "I'm going to do this at exactly the level I want. I don't care."
- "I'm good at justifying my behavior."
- "I haven't seen any consequences yet."
- "I don't believe the consequences I have seen are a result of my current behavior."
- "My results are due to bad luck and bad DNA, so there is no reason for me to change." (For the record, only 2 - 5% of disease is DNA related)
- "I don't wanna!"

You would never accept your spouse cheating on you in moderation. We don't tolerate someone stealing cars in moderation. Drug users die using in moderation. Why do we all nod in agreement when someone engages in unhealthy eating "in moderation?"

If you want to continue to engage in a behavior that is less than healthy, it's 100% your choice. But make that choice with your eyes wide open, recognizing and accepting the risks. Don't turn a blind eye and lie to yourself that it's perfectly fine because it's "in moderation."

In the very least, don't lie to us. It makes my psychologist brain want to explode.

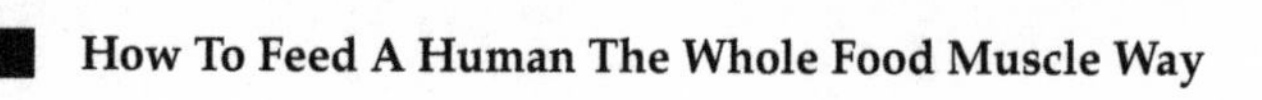

When Food = Happiness (Addiction)

Dr. Joel Fuhrman, President of the Nutritional Research Foundation, has said that if a human being is overweight, they have a food addiction. We know that might be hard to hear. But bear with us. Humans are not designed to be immensely overweight. We have internal mechanisms that should tell us "hey, you've had enough." But those mechanisms have been hijacked by the food industry. Big Food spends millions of dollars studying exactly how food changes our brain chemistry and how to make their products as pleasurable as possible. The more pleasure (the brain chemical dopamine) someone gets from a product, the more of it they will eat and the more money the company makes. And when food companies are questioned about creating addicting products, they shrug and say our heath isn't their responsibility. They aren't forcing anyone to eat their products.

We have heard some pretty shocking things when talking to people about food. "Eating steak is my one joy in life." "I'd rather be happy than healthy." "I'd rather die young eating what I want." These are sad examples of how people use food for pleasure (which is not the same as happiness) rather than fuel.

Pleasure versus happiness

Pleasure is a short-term gratification. Sex, drugs and yes, food, cause a rush of dopamine, which feels really good. Calorie-dense foods loaded with fat, sugar and salt are going to create a much bigger rush than say, cabbage. But foods loaded with nutrients (like cabbage) create long-term happiness. Unfortunately, humans get addicted to the short-term hit and pass up the opportunity for happiness.

Because of the quick pleasure hit we get from processed foods, we are prone to using it as a reward and to cover unhappiness. Going through a messy break up? Add ice cream (fat, sugar, salt) and wine! Tough day at the office? Oh, look. The same prescription applies. Get a promotion? The same again. Having a birthday, get engaged, close a big deal, going to have an awkward meeting with your in-laws? Bring on the fat, sugar, salt and alcohol. Did your kid do something great? Everything but the alcohol!

As humans, we are taught from a very young age to use food as an emotional regulator. Why feel your emotions and deal with them when you can just cover them up with food?

There is no greater evidence of food addiction in the general public than when we suggest people stop eating cheese (see the **Cheese May be the Death of You** chapter). "But I LOVE cheese!" they whine. Yes. Yes, you do. Because you are addicted. If the idea of giving up a certain food product makes you actively convulse with fear, you can be pretty sure you have an addiction. Most people like to call it a "craving," so we will collude in that little story for now.

Overcoming food cravings

Food cravings are a real thing. Anyone who tells you otherwise is either SUPER lucky or lying and our bet is on lying. But how do you know if something is a craving? If you think, "Hmm, I would like to eat something," you know you're likely hungry. On the other hand, if you think, "Hmm, I would like to eat THAT thing" and nothing else really sounds good, you can safely bet it's a craving.

Are food cravings always bad?

We don't think of cravings as necessarily good / bad. Your body is likely trying to tell you something. Unfortunately, most of us crave foods that are not very healthy (loaded with fat, sugar and salt) and we don't do a good job of figuring out what our body is actually trying to say so we can fix it. That's why we get the munchies (not drug-related). Our body wants nutrients, but we know we've had enough calories. So, we just randomly start putting addictive, industry- created snacks in our mouths that do nothing for our nutrient needs.

> ***Humans are not designed to be immensely overweight. We have internal mechanisms that should tell us "hey, you've had enough." But those mechanisms have been hijacked by the food industry.***

What causes food cravings?

- **Lack of sleep –** If you aren't getting enough good quality shut-eye, your body is going to be looking for quick-fix energy. Nothing works better for that than fat, sugar and salt. Throw in some caffeine and you can continue to ignore the call of your bed. Study after study shows that most adults are sleep deprived. It is highly unlikely that you are an exception.

- **Lack of water –** Being dehydrated can cause cravings for food. Drink more water.

- **Lack of nutrients –** We've talked a lot about how the Standard American Diet/Western Diet that most people eat doesn't have nearly enough nutrients in it. Your cells could be starving. Your evolution says, "Find something calorie dense" because it makes the mistake of assuming that calories = nutrition. For example, sugar addiction is your body screaming for nutrients, but we mistake it for wanting energy (calories). We, and our clients, have found that the desire for sugar (especially in the evenings) goes away when breakfast and lunch are low-calorie density and high-nutritional density foods (real foods, not supplements or fake food-like products).

- **Lack of bulk (fiber) –** If you've eaten enough calories but still crave something it could be that you're not getting enough fiber in your diet to make you feel full and feed your gut bacteria.

- **Unhappy gut flora –** The human gut is an amazing place. Healthy bacteria can reduce inflammation, make you feel better and generally keep things humming along. But unhappy gut bacteria can make life miserable, including creating sugar cravings.

- **Emotions –** Eating to cover emotions is often passed off as cravings. But really, it's the chemical rush you're looking for.

- **Habit –** Pavlovian eating. We mentioned this in the **I Know I Should Eat Better, But...** chapter. Eating due to an outside stimulus is like a smoker who smokes just because they are in the car. Habit plus addiction creates a powerful craving!

- **Social setting –** Sometimes a craving is just about where you are and who you're hanging with. When junk food is easily available, such as at a party, it can feel almost impossible to not have some.

What can you do about cravings?

The "easy" answers are: get enough sleep, stay hydrated, eat real food that feeds your cells, eat whole foods that have fiber in them, avoid strong emotions, address all your eating triggers and don't be social. Okay, the last three are a bit much to ask. But the rest of them are certainly doable. And if you do the rest, you'll be more likely to resist stuffing yourself with fat, sugar and salt just because you feel bad, have a Pavlovian response to a trigger or are out with friends.

Keep a craving calendar

Another thing you can do is start keeping a cravings calendar. When do you crave what? Do you have triggers? How often do you give in? Write it down. Color code it if that helps you (adding color to make patterns easy to see is always good for me). The more you know about what is happening, the easier it is to do something about it.

Disconnect a time or an activity from eating

Cravings are often triggered by outside forces, having nothing to do with hunger, the need for calories or even because your body needed a specific nutrient. Your best opportunity to not give into a craving is realizing you are having one. Asking yourself these questions before you start eating can help you catch a craving and give you the opportunity to stop it in its tracks:

- **Am I actually hungry?** That question is harder to answer than you'd think. Because your brain is all too happy to say "Yes!" If you aren't happy eating an apple or broccoli, you aren't hungry, you have a craving.

- **When did I last eat?** If the answer is less than 3-4 hours ago and you ate enough of something nutrient dense, it's likely you don't need another meal's worth of calories of fat, sugar and salt right now. (**Side note:** you never NEED a fatty / sugary / salty snack).

- **Why am I choosing to eat this?** Too often we don't think about the food choice we are making. It is simply a habit triggered by what is going on around us. If we can catch ourselves eating without thinking, we have a chance to make a choice. Whether it is healthy or not, at least we are making a conscious choice. (See below for more on why we make the choices we make.)

- **Is there a whole-plant food I could eat now?** Whole-plant foods such as fruits, veggies and starches are high bulk and low calories. Their volume fills our stomachs so we can't eat any more before eating more calories than we can burn. Replacing the animal-based proteins, fats and the junk-food carbs you eat out of habit with fresh or frozen fruits and vegetables, whole grains, beans, and plant starches (yes, even rice and potatoes) will make you think about what you are eating. That's a good thing!

Your best opportunity to not give into a craving is realizing you are having one.

All that said, occasionally it's not a huge deal. It's not the exception that causes the problem, it's the every day. Sometimes (every few months at most) I give in to a craving and I have a chocolate chip cookie. And you know what? IT IS AMAZING! I really enjoy it because it is a rare treat. Now, I know that after I give in, I'm going to have to deal with wanting another and another. So, I only buy a two pack. That's it. No more cookies in the house. If I want a cookie, I have to make a point to go to the store to get it. Most of the time when I think about a cookie, I don't have the time or the desire to go get one. For me, rule number one for fighting cravings – don't have cookies in the house!

How do you choose the foods you eat?

Do you know WHY you choose the foods you eat? When we ask this question, the answers usually range from "I like it" (taste) to "it's easy" (convenience). And while those are the easy answers, we think there is a lot more going into it that we don't consider until we start reflecting on changing what we eat.

Culture – What you like, what tastes good to you, is much more about how you've trained your taste buds than anything else. And your taste buds have been trained by the culture where you grew up. How much fat, sugar and salt you like in your food depends on what part of the world you spent your formative years.

Media/Advertising – Have you ever been sitting in front of the TV and suddenly thought, "Hmmm, pizza sounds good?" If you can honestly answer "no," we would be shocked. They don't run TV ads for the fun of it. We are bombarded every day by food ads. They are even on social media. Every time you see gooey cheese dripping from pasta or potatoes or whatever, you can bet your brain is storing that information away for later.

Cost – Maybe you think that cost doesn't really drive your food choices. But if you've ever thought "organic is so expensive" or this fast food lunch is only $5, cost is part of your food choice process. We understand that everyone is on a budget. We are not saying you shouldn't be. We are just saying we need to be aware if cost is a contributing factor in our choices.

Habit – If you watch our Facebook Lives (*www.FB.com/RnRJourneyToHealth*) you've heard me talk about Pavlovian eating. It's the eating we do because it's time to eat, we always have popcorn at the movies, or even turkey at Thanksgiving (which is also cultural).

Easy – Yep. Convenience is really a thing. But it's not just, "this food is here" like at an office lunch. Unconsciously we also think, "Do I need a fork to eat this?" "Do I have to sit down?" "How hard is this to chew?" We had someone tell us that eating plants was hard because they didn't have time to chew it (that sparked a whole conversation about believing that feeding ourselves is an inconvenient annoyance).

Many times, dare we say MOST of the time, what you choose to eat has nothing to do with hunger and worse, nutrition never crosses your minds. But let's say you're ready to change that. Where do you start?

Here are a couple of quick tips:

Notice when you make a food choice. Paying attention is half the battle.

- Ask yourself WHY you are making (or made) the choice. Identifying triggers gives you the opportunity to change.

- Tell yourself a story. What would it look like if you made a different choice? Pay attention to the story you tell. Is it heartache and pain or joy and happiness? The story you tell about food is important.

- Look at your cost/benefit analysis. That sounds complicated but it's not. What are you telling yourself about your food choices and your health (this is part of your story)?

- Don't get caught up in all-or-nothing thinking – There seems to be a prevailing belief that you either have to eat 100% healthy or throw your hands in the air and give up. This is not a pass/fail class. If you can average an A- or B+ or better you're doing really well! (Of course, being the high performer that you are, we know you're looking at that A/A+ thinking, "Oh yeah. I can totally do that!")

Try thinking about it using this scale:

- A+ = Whole-plant foods. Stuff that looks like it came out of the ground (sweet potatoes, fruits, veggies, grains, etc.)
- A = Minimally processed plant foods (steel cut oats)
- B+ = Processed plant foods (whole wheat breads and pastas.) Russ' Rustic Bread falls here
- B- = Junk "health" foods (veggie burgers)
- C = refined carbs (foodstuffs in packages without animal products and oil)
- C- = oil, fried plants (French fries)
- D = Animal protein (meat, including fish)
- D- = Dairy and eggs
- F = Fried animal products and processed meat (yes, bacon is an F)

The unfortunate thing is eating the Standard American Diet (SAD) will give you an average of a D, D+ at best! Being junk-food vegan, you might get a B- or a C. We know you can do better than that. Let's get those averages up by being more aware of what we are eating on a daily basis!

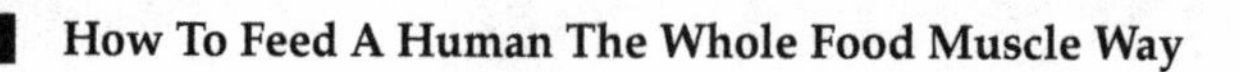

Overcoming Self-Sabotage

"I had a stressful day, so I deserve…"

"I lost a few pounds so it's okay if I have…"

"I exercise so I can eat whatever I want."

"I gained a few pounds and I'm disheartened so…"

"I already ate xyz unhealthy thing, so who cares what I eat now?"

"I just need to eat healthy until (insert event or weight goal). After that I can eat what I want."

Do any of those sound familiar? If so, you likely have an inner saboteur. But that doesn't mean you are destined to failure. I've never met anyone (including myself) who didn't have a self-sabotaging streak. The key is to recognize it and manage it. It is part of who you are, so you can't kick it to the curb. You're stuck with it on this ride we call life. But you don't have to let it drive or give directions.

What causes self-sabotage?

That is the subject of whole books. But the short answer is, the voice in your head that tells you you can't, you shouldn't, you'll fail, you always fail, don't try and if you succeed, that it was luck. Every negative thing you believe about yourself is your inner saboteur speaking.

Why do we self-sabotage?

Most of us have someone or several someones who we loved and looked up to who were our "voice of reason." "Don't try that. You might get hurt."

"Don't do that. You'll fail and look stupid." "Don't pat yourself on the back too hard." "That success was just luck." Self-sabotage gets passed from person to person like a virus. And inevitably when someone tells us not to try something and we do it anyway, we sometimes fail (that's what happens when you're learning). But the person uses it as evidence that they were right and our inner saboteur is born. It doesn't take much to grow an inner saboteur. Trying new things. Doing foolish things as a child. Being teased, made fun of and ostracized. Most of us have a healthy inner saboteur by the time we are in grade school.

But finding a place to put the blame and solving the problem isn't the same thing. So, let's keep moving.

What is the voice in your head saying?

Do you actually listen to the words? It's unlikely unless you've written them down. Your inner saboteur communicates mostly in feelings (guilt, shame, regret, disappointment, fear, etc.). And feelings don't get translated into words unless we need to communicate them to someone else. Unfortunately, if they aren't words, your logical brain can't process them. The feelings just swirl around in your emotional brain and get bigger and more intimidating.

What to do about self-sabotage

As silly as it sounds, the first thing I recommend you do is give your inner saboteur a name. I call mine Harry-ette. She was given that name 25+ years ago, before I ever took a single college class (I had no idea it was a real psychology thing to do). I named her because I wanted to be able to recognize her voice and tell her to shut up!

Tips for naming your saboteur:

- Don't choose a popular name. You don't want to end up working with or being friends with someone with the same name as your inner critic.
- Don't choose a name of someone you disliked as a kid. There is too much emotional baggage attached to a name that belongs to someone you know now or knew before.
- Do choose a name that feels right to you. Take your time. It takes some people several days to come up with a name.
- Do learn to recognize his/her voice and attach his/her name to it.
- Do share your inner critic's name with your coach or therapist (if you have one). It will help you discuss your self-sabotaging habits in a more productive way.

Start to pay attention to what your inner saboteur is saying. You might find it helpful to journal about it (that will allow your logical brain to be involved). Do you agree with that voice? Do you disagree? Which of you is running your life? Those can be tough questions to answer on your own. Working with a qualified professional can make a world of difference. Don't let your saboteur convince you you're not worth it, don't deserve to have someone help you or that you can't afford it.

If you'd like my help putting your inner saboteur in the backseat, send an email to Health@RnRJourney.com and let's chat.

Look out for "irrelevant decisions" Every day we make micro-decisions that feel like they have no meaning in the grand scheme of our lives. But when we look at them closely, we realize they can be our downfall. Pay attention to choices that, on the surface, don't feel like they are related to your success in any way. Examples might include:

- Deciding to hang out with that person who always says, "You can have this unhealthy thing this one time, certainly."
- Calling the person who tells you, "You look fine. You don't need to be worried about eating healthy."
- Being "too busy" to eat before a meeting where you know there will be pizza.
- Being "too busy" to plan healthy meals.
- Wearing sweats/leggings or other stretchy clothing ALL the time.
- Telling an unsupportive friend or family member about the changes you are trying to make.

Little choices like these give our inner skeptic fuel to throw back at us later. When you listen to the voice in your head, pay attention to what he/she is using against you. It will help you identify where you are making "irrelevant decisions" that are hurting your success.

Are you afraid to succeed?

If you are like most people, and absolutely like most high performers, you very quickly answered that question with a resounding, "NO!" Maybe I shouldn't have asked if "you" are afraid to succeed, but if your inner saboteur is afraid to succeed. In that case the response might be a quiet, guilt-laden "maybe." That's okay. We can work with that.

Ruminating (letting it just churn over and over in your head) about something is never helpful, even though inner critics love to do it. But there is a game you can play with yourself called "catastrophication" (at least that was what my psychology prof. called it). Take the time to go to the absolute worst-case (or best-case depending on how you look at it) scenario. What if you succeed? Like really, really succeed? What are the worst things and the best things that could happen?

Every day we make micro-decisions that feel like they have no meaning in the grand scheme of our lives. But when we look at them closely, we realize they can be our downfall.

"My friends will hate me because I'll be healthy."

"I won't be able to go out with my boyfriend because he likes to eat wings."

"I'll be the weird one at business lunches."

"People will think I think I'm better than they are."

"My family won't come over for dinner because they won't like the food I make."

Really go to town. Get all that stuff, crazy or otherwise, out of your head. You can't process it if it's stuck swirling around in your emotional brain.

You can also use this process for a fear of failure. "What if I try and fail?" Again, get anything and everything that comes up down on paper.

Once you have all the things written down (so your logical brain can see them), go through them one by one and ask yourself, "Really, how likely is this thing to happen?" Usually it's pretty unlikely. But be honest with yourself. Then ask yourself, "Okay, if this happened, then what would I do?" And come up with a plan. If your fears involve other people like several of the examples above, talk to those people. You might be surprised how supportive they are.

This process does a couple of things. One, it lets your logical brain say, "That's never going to happen so I can stop thinking about it." Two, if by some odd chance it does happen, "I now have a plan to address it so I can stop worrying about it."

This game works for both the fear of failure and the fear of success. But it only works if you write it down. Just thinking about it might make the situation worse. Your emotional brain and self-saboteur aren't going to solve anything between them. Your logical brain needs to be involved. It can also be helpful to work through things with a qualified and caring professional.

Self-sabotaging is a real and challenging issue. But with some focused effort, your "Harry-ette" will learn to ride quietly in the backseat on your life journey, or in the very least, you'll be able to just roll your eyes at him/her and keep making progress towards your goals. See the next chapter for more on that.

When Family and Friends Derail You

I went back and forth about including this chapter because there is so much individual nuance in personal relationships. Such as why people make the choices they make and how they are supported or not by the people around them. In the end, I decided to touch on a few of the most common challenges and provide general tips. With that said, if you are in a situation where your significant other, parent, family or friend is actively trying to sabotage your success, send us an email at Health@RnRJourney.com and let's schedule time to have a conversation about your unique situation.

They love you into failure

When someone loves you, they want you to be happy. Many of us associate happiness with food (but that's actually pleasure). In an effort to make you happy, they might buy you things you don't want to eat, like the guy who buys his wife chocolate on Valentine's Day, gets in trouble for it and then his feelings are hurt (cue: relationship drama). We even have this happen to us. I happen to LOVE chocolate chip cookies (the ones that are really unhealthy; loaded with sugar, butter and eggs). Every once in a while I'll say, "I'd really like a cookie." Inevitably Russ' reply is along the lines of, "If you want a cookie, I'll take you to get a cookie." Sigh. "Yes. I want a cookie. No. I don't want to go get a cookie."

I totally understand why that is confusing. Sometimes I just want to SAY I want a cookie, because I REALLY do! But I also know they aren't healthy and once I have one it's going to turn the cravings on and I'm going to want them more often. I don't actually want to HAVE a cookie.

(For the record, I did have two full-on "awful-for-me" chocolate chip cookies on my birthday. And I enjoyed them very much. Thank you, Russ!)

If this is happening to you, there are a couple of things you can do:

- Explain how much you appreciate their desire to make you happy.
- Suggest other ways they can show they love you.
- Ask them for ideas of other ways to show caring and love.
- Brainstorm things you can do together to take the place of unhealthy treats.
- Tell them my chocolate chip cookie story.

It's not the once or twice a year that's a problem. It's the every week or more. If you aren't sure how often you are giving in to "I-love-you-food," start keeping a calendar. There is nothing that will highlight a bad habit faster than writing it down and seeing the pattern in ink.

They are emotionally afraid

This can be a little more challenging to identify. If someone has gotten comfortable with you as an unhealthy person and now you're on a path to being healthy, they might be scared. Maybe they're scared you'll force them to change. Afraid you'll leave them. Worried it will change your relationship, or even scared of something they can't identify.

Having a conversation about this can be hard. Your loved one might say they support you and want you to succeed. But then they engage in actions that suggest otherwise (bringing unhealthy foods into the house, wanting to go out to eat all the time, criticizing you, teasing you in public).

In private, when you are able to be calm and rational, ask about the disparity between what they say and their actions. Don't accuse them of anything. Simply ask them why that is happening and listen to what they say. Some people are going to deflect and defend. Perhaps you can say, "I know you want to support me. I'd like to share some ways you can do that."

This conversation is always uniquely personal and how it goes depends on the relationship you have with the person, your past communications and how safe each of you feels emotionally. If they legitimately want you to succeed and just have a few things to work through to be able to best support you, you're in a great place. Someone who loves you and is willing to try can always learn. If you would like support in having or creating this conversation, send us an email at Health@RnRJourney.com.

> ***If someone has gotten comfortable with you as an unhealthy person and now you're on a path to being healthy, they might be scared.***

They are emotionally abusive about your choice

Sometimes we have to get together with the people who know our buttons and love pushing them on purpose. I have often wondered why we do that to ourselves. But it is often expected and so we do (I have stopped doing things that result in emotional abuse just because they are expected. But that is a deeper conversation than I can have in this chapter). The best we can do is gather our wits and our best conflict-resolution skills and smile.

I have written other books on conflict resolution and it boils down to one thing; you get to control you, your emotions and your physical space. As long as you keep your head (logical brain) and don't let your emotional brain takeover, you will be in control.

A couple of quick tips for doing that:

Recognize when your body is telling you things aren't okay. We all have a physical "tell." That thing our body does when we feel hurt, threatened or unsafe. Maybe your stomach sinks or clutches or maybe your chest gets tight or your neck and shoulders clench. Whatever your tell is, pay attention to it. When it happens, you have the briefest of moments for your logical brain to be involved. Miss it and you'll just have to hang on for the ride as your emotional brain takes over (like that time you said things that were true, but not kind or the time you couldn't think of a good response until an hour later) and everyone leaves hurt, angry or worse.

Expect the best, but be prepared for the crazy. Have a canned answer that you can just continue to use. Depending on how snarky you want to be, here are some ideas:

"This choice is working for me for now."

"I've done the research and am really excited about this."

"Fortunately, I am an adult and get to make my own choices/mistakes."

"I appreciate your caring. That isn't a conversation I am willing to have."

"It's a personal choice and I'm not interested in having to defend it."

"I'm here to enjoy time with the family / friends. Let's stick with topics that make that possible."

"My answer hasn't changed since the last time we talked about it."

"Ugh, that's an awkward topic for the dinner table."

"By all means, let's find a divisive topic so we can all leave unhappy."

One of the most common things that will cause get-togethers to crash and burn is too much alcohol. Be aware how much you drink (it's not healthy anyway). Your logical brain can't be involved if you're buzzed (or worse). And if things deteriorate as people get drunk, plan on saying your goodbyes and leaving before it gets out of hand.

There is always that one person (hopefully, only one) who takes great joy in razzing, teasing and generally making people the butt of their jokes. If you say anything, their response will be, "You're too thin-skinned" or "You never could take a joke."

First let's be clear, it is never your responsibility to have thick skin so someone can cut you and laugh while you bleed. It's not cool and it's not okay for someone to purposefully be harmful or mean. You have a spectrum of options from laughing awkwardly, rolling your eyes, ignoring them or pushing back. Decide what strategy you want to employ ahead of time and guard your heart from their arrows.

Don't revert to old roles. Too often when we are around people we've known forever, we go back to familiar, unhealthy roles. You are not a child. You are not trapped without choices. You do not have to put up with unhealthy behavior just to be "polite." That is important enough that I'm going to write it again. You do NOT have to put up with unhealthy behavior just to be polite. You can choose to use healthy coping patterns. Walk away. Go to the bathroom. Make a phone call (Not to complain. Just to change the energy). Talk to someone else. Think about what a great story you'll have to tell later. Have a funny story to tell. Talk about sports or something that interests you. Ask questions about how everyone is and what's going on with them. I have found that most inappropriate comments/questions happen when there is a lull in the conversation and someone wants attention.

Don't fan the flames, but also don't feel you have to be the fire department. Depending on your role, you could find yourself in a heated, verbal battle about something that isn't even your issue (I have found myself in this role with total strangers!). Sometimes a simple, "That's not cool" or "That wasn't nice" or "Let's not put people on the spot" or the ever popular, "Awkward!" is enough to cut the tension and have things move on.

How to deal with comments about how you eat

You might hear things like, "It's Thanksgiving! Surely you can have some turkey" or "That isn't a healthy way to eat" or "You can't get enough protein from plants" or "Your diet isn't working." "You're still fat" or any number of other ugly, uninformed, rude, hurtful, mean and just wrong comments.

First – don't argue. No one is going to have their mind changed about how they eat while tucking into a full-on fat, sugar, salt, animal product orgy. Just keep saying, "This is the choice I've made for my health and I feel great." And leave it at that.

If they try to pressure, bully or trick you – "Peer pressure? Really? We aren't in junior high. Certainly, we are adult enough to respect each other's choices."

If someone just won't leave you alone you could say, "You might be right. But I'm going to do this anyway." Sometimes you have to just let someone be wrong because they feel so strongly they are right. Some people are afraid to learn anything new because it means changing what they know and the truth they are comfortable with. As annoying as that is, you don't have to let it affect your long-term health by eating something you know isn't ideal for your health.

Setting Yourself up to Succeed (Developing Grit)

As a high performer you have likely heard of and even have grit. Most of us who are able to achieve things in life usually do. But you might not have considered how you can use it to succeed at improving your health and longevity. If you don't have as much grit as you wish you had, don't worry. This chapter is going to give you everything you need to know to get started.

What is grit?

Grit is the ability to keep going, keep trying and continuing to make progress. The willingness to set a goal and work towards it, even if that means pivoting the path you take to get there. Athletes, entrepreneurs, successful business people and anyone who has achieved success through work, persistence and determination have shown they have grit. Many perceive working towards their goals and dealing with the inevitable setbacks as thrilling, and believe it makes success sweeter to have had to work for it.

Grit can be a somewhat fickle trait. It is possible to have it in one situation, such as being an athlete, but have it disappear in another area like, giving a public talk. Both are performance-based, so you'd think grit would show up in both places. But there are underlying emotional challenges that can bury our grit. I believe that is what happens when high achievers struggle with making and sticking to their health goals, particularly when it comes to changing their diet.

Breaking the idea of grit down into its component parts will allow you to apply it to any big goal you have (including your health).

How are people with grit different?

People with grit see their goals and plans as giving direction to their lives. Having things they want to achieve, even things other people think are too big and too crazy, gives meaning to their lives. For people who haven't developed their grit yet, goals, especially big ones, can seem like overwhelming drudgery, things they HAVE to do rather than things they GET to do.

Grit is the ability to keep going, keep trying and continuing to make progress. The willingness to set a goal and work towards it, even if that means pivoting the path you take to get there.

Those possessing grit also realize that any great achievement is just a collection of mostly mundane, even boring, tasks. TV, movies and every available entertainment has taught us life should be exciting and thrilling at all times and that being bored is a bad thing. Those of us who succeed at big things realize it usually just means consistently doing lots of relatively uninteresting things. I say that about my workouts. None of them are overly impressive or hard anymore. I go, do a workout and leave. No pain, struggle or grit required. But I go five days a week. Yes, it's boring sometimes. But that persistence means I continuously have a healthy body.

This idea of repeatedly doing mundane tasks to achieve big goals can also be applied to diet. Consider things like finding a new recipe to try, learning a new health tidbit, deciding to bring your lunch and having foods that fit into the Whole Food Muscle Way in the house. None of those things by themselves are interesting, earth-shattering or even hard. But done consistently over time, even when you aren't excited about it, leads to achieving long-term goals like better health, a healthier weight and even longevity.

Grit is not a talent

The ability to wake up the next day and try again is not something some people were lucky enough to be born with and others are just out of luck. Most things that people consider "talents" are actually years of focused practice, failure, get feedback and repeat. Sure, there are some people who are born able to play Mozart or are a bit more naturally athletic than others (My brother Ben is one of those unbelievably athletic people). But for the vast majority of us, being good at something means we cared enough to learn and work at it over a long period of time.

Let's say you want to develop the skill of feeding yourself the ideal human diet to achieve better health and weight. No one is born with the ability to do that. It's learned. The first thing to do is gain knowledge of what is the ideal diet for humans. Great, this book explains that.

Once you have that knowledge, you'll have to decide how you're going to apply it to your life. That's going to take some effort. Maybe you'll need to develop some cooking skills. You might need to rethink your path through the grocery store. Possibly get a good chef's knife and cutting board? Whatever small changes you need to make.

Now that you have the knowledge and a few new skills, you can start putting them into practice (yep, more effort). Sometimes it will work out well (pat yourself on the back for those) and other times you'll get the feedback that something didn't work. That's okay too; it's just part of the achievement process.

There is a saying in the sports world, "What is hard today will someday be your warm-up." Interestingly, that is only true if you do the "hard" thing today. Fortunately, nothing we are talking about here is actually hard. It's just different than you're used to.

Dealing with the frustration of starting

It is really annoying to try to do something you can't do yet. The negative voice in our head (insert the name of your inner saboteur here) tells us we are lousy at this and we'll never get better. It's frustrating, uncomfortable and even emotionally painful to struggle. And it's easy to just say, "I can't" and go back to the easy way that we know. But being willing to deal with the frustration of learning is at the foundation of success.

Let me share an example of a time I wasn't willing to overcome the frustration of being a beginner and because of it, I can't do something now:

When I was in eighth grade, my dad, a high school music teacher, took me with him to a jazz festival in Reno, Nevada where his school band was competing. One evening, after the competition, everyone decided to go bowling. I had never bowled. But since the whole band and all the chaperones where going, I didn't have a choice.

I was AWFUL! I don't think I bowled a single ball that didn't end up in the gutter. As you know, high schoolers can be merciless. Not only did they tease me that night, they continued to tease me for the rest of the trip and the ride home (I was the teacher's kid, after all).

To this day, I have NEVER picked up another bowling ball. My inner eighth grader is still mortified. Now, I am a reasonable athlete. My eye-hand coordination is good and I am coachable. It is a pretty safe bet that, given the willingness to overcome my frustration and embarrassment (and assuming I had the desire and opportunity), I could have become a tolerable bowler.

We'll never know because I allowed the shame and embarrassment of being a beginner stop me before I even started. Don't let that be the story of your health journey. The consequences are much higher than not being able to bowl. Just because you're bad at something the first time you try it doesn't mean you can't do it. You just need useful feedback, practice and a little perseverance.

Speaking of feedback...

You can use someone else's grit to achieve your goals. Read that line again. You can use someone else's grit to help achieve your goals. Here's how:

Work with a coach or accountability partner or join a group (like the Whole Food Muscle Club *www.WholeFoodMuscle.com/bookdiscount*) of people all trying to achieve a similar goal. Having someone to talk to who believes in you will help shore up your grit when you want to give up, particularly if they are also a high achiever. People who have a history of succeeding are really good at cheerleading another person's success.

BUT (notice that is a big but), your support needs to come from someone who can give you useful, productive feedback that you can actually use to get better. You might be tempted to just talk to a friend and assume they will be able to give you feedback and support your grit. People who don't understand giving useful feedback will often give critical feedback (just tell you what they see as wrong with what you are doing). They aren't able to give you any tips, suggestions or ideas on how to tweak your approach to move closer to your goal.

An example of this is a boss who gives feedback like, "I don't like it." Great. What are you supposed to do with that? In your health journey someone might just commiserate with you about how hard change is. No one needs help wallowing. Both of those types of feedback are likely to lead to you feeling discouraged, not encouraged, and aren't going to bolster your grit.

(Part of our big WHY in creating the Whole Food Muscle Club was to let you use our grit and the collective grit of the community. There is step-by-step guidance and support. You can share your successes, challenges and suggestions, and even chat with other Whole Food Muscle members. Plus, our monthly Ask Us Anything Q&A sessions where you get direct access to us. Ask your questions live or email them to us prior to the event (Health@RnRJourney.com). If you can't make it live, the replay is posted in the members section so you can watch it at your convenience.

You can use someone else's grit to achieve your goals.

We are very fortunate because we have each other to lean on when our individual grit runs thin (except when Russ wants to buy me cookies). You want someone who can support your success. Look for someone who can help you:

- Clearly define your goal

- Break it down into manageable, doable parts
- Believe you can
- Support full concentration and effort
- Talk through challenges
- Learn from slip-ups
- Get immediate and informative feedback
- Suggest useful tweaks
- Support repetition
- Celebrate success (not with eating junk)

As an athlete, I had a mantra: Practice, Perform, Evaluate, Adjust, Repeat. Think about the practice part as learning about this new way of feeding yourself. Perform is actually doing it (clearly), Evaluate – how is it working for you. Adjust – tweak things to make it work better or more successfully and move the process towards your goal. Repeat – I don't need to explain that one.

The one place the sports analogy breaks down is in the competition. Your health and longevity are not a competition with anyone. When you compare yourself to someone else, you are using them as a measuring stick. If you compared yourself to someone who had been successfully following the Whole Food Muscle Way for many years, you'd deem yourself a failure. If instead, you compared your eating to a college student surviving on beer, pizza and ramen noodles, you'd pat yourself on the back as a raging success. You didn't change. Only your comparative data did. Your only competition is you. Did you do better today than you did yesterday? If yes, great! Keep doing it. If no, look at what happened and how can you make tomorrow better.

You can move a mountain with a teaspoon if you are willing to commit to working on it every day. We bet your goal isn't that daunting.

Some Logistics

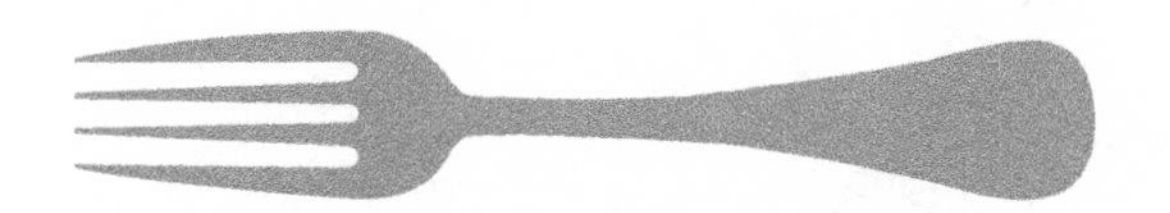

How Losing Weight Works

There is a lot of confusion around what weight loss or weight gain really are. We recently went out for vegetable sushi and I gained three pounds! Someone posted recently that they fasted for 22 hours and lost four pounds (they were so excited). Another post proudly announced losing a pound that week. One complained they had been "very strict" on their diet and hadn't lost any weight in ten days. Yet another poster was stuck for a few weeks and then whoosh — they lost two or three pounds almost overnight. The human body doesn't gain or lose body fat that quickly. So, what is going on?

In my case the extra three pounds was water retention caused by the sodium in the soy sauce enjoyed with veggie sushi. That weight was gone in about three days. Too much sodium in the body can be dangerous, so we offset that risk by holding onto water. This water weight is stored in your tissue until your body can rid itself of the excess sodium and believes the threat is passed. It's not weight as in fat; it's just water. Stay well hydrated; don't take in so much sodium and the issue goes away.

What about losing four pounds in a day? There are a couple of things at play when fasting, particularly for someone whose body has not adjusted to fasting.

One – people often allow themselves to get dehydrated when they fast. Too little water will cause weight loss just like retaining too much results in weight gain.

Two – when fasting, your body is going to burn the glycogen that is stored in your muscles. That can be up to two pounds just in glycogen, plus the four to six pounds of water stored with it. Your body will burn fat when fasting. BUT you won't notice that on the scale the same day (see why below).

Three – your body uses the break it gets from processing food during fasting to do some housekeeping, reducing inflammation and sending broken and dead cells out with the trash (we have read that the human body replaces 50,000 cells a second – this wasn't a peer-reviewed scientific source and who knows how they actually measure such things. But it's interesting to consider.) Between dehydration, glycogen burn and inflammation reduction, losing four pounds while fasting isn't shocking. But don't be surprised when most of it comes back in a day or two. (**Note:** We are usually down two-ish pounds on fasting days. Most likely this is glycogen that is replaced the next day when we eat.)

Your body will burn fat when fasting. BUT you won't notice that on the scale the same day.

The whoosh effect. Yep, that is a real term. We both experienced it during our weight loss journey. We thought we had plateaued because our weight wasn't changing and then, whoosh –two to three pounds overnight. It happens because as your body burns fat out of a fat cell, it replaces it with water as a holding spot for fat later. When the cell becomes 100% water and your body realizes, "Oh I don't need this cell for fat" it pulls all the water out and the cell goes flat. The sudden drop in weight is your body emptying fat cells of that water. If your weight plateaus and then you suddenly lose a couple of pounds, it's fat weight you likely burned a week or more ago. Your body is just catching up. Don't worry about it or try to change it. It's normal and healthy.

Losing or gaining weight isn't about the number on the scale today compared to the number yesterday or tomorrow. It's about the trend over a week or a month. If you're geeky like me, you can create an Excel graph with a trend line. Feed your cells nutritious, fiber-rich, whole-plant foods, move your body and you will find and maintain your ideal body weight easily.

To get an idea of what your optimum weight for health and longevity is, read the next chapter, **How Much Should I Weigh?**

Losing or gaining weight isn't about the number on the scale today compared to the number yesterday or tomorrow. It's about the trend over a week or a month.

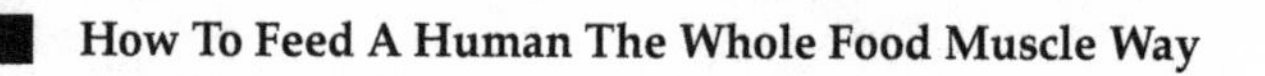

How Much Should I Weigh?

Weight it a funny thing. It's just a number on a scale. But it is often how we judge ourselves. For so many, that number is what determines if they feel good or bad about themselves. We had one woman tell us she doesn't weigh herself because if the number is "good" she uses it as an excuse to reward herself with unhealthy food and if it is "bad" it is a reason to give up and binge eat.

Weight is one point of data, useful certainly, but not the be-all-and-end-all. You likely think you know if you are within a healthy weight or not. But we have discovered most people have no clue what a healthy-weight human looks like. It is shocking how many of our clients (and we) have been skinny-shamed. Told by friends, loved ones, acquaintances and even perfect strangers that we are "too thin," "look gaunt," "shouldn't lose any more weight," or asked in a hushed tone, "Are you sick?"

Here are a few resources you can use to determine what your optimum weight is for health and longevity and to ease the minds of your loved ones that you are, indeed, on the right track. Know that most concerned individuals are used to seeing people carrying more than a few extra pounds, so they have no idea what a healthy weight human looks like and they don't know what they are talking about.

BMI

There are hundreds of BMI (body mass index) calculators out there. We would suggest you simply Google one and plug your numbers in. If you want to go old-school and calculate it by hand, this is the formula: BMI =

kg/m^2 (your weight in **kilograms** divided by your height in meters squared).

Convert pounds to kilograms: pounds x 0.453592

Convert inches to meters: inches x 0.0254

Example for a person 5'6" weighing 165 pounds:

165 x 0.453592 = 74.84268kg

66 x 0.0254 = 1.6764m

$74.84268 / 1.6764^2 = 74.84268 / 2.84031696 = 26.63$ (overweight)

(But really, just use Google)

BMI tells you if you fall in line with what "they" (whoever they are in this case) deem normal; which is generally accepted has healthy.

- 18.5-24.9 = normal
- 25-29.9 = overweight
- 30 or greater = obese
- 40 or greater or 35 + obesity-related health conditions = morbidly obese.

BMI is a SUPER rough data point. The drawbacks of using BMI include: no variation for men/women, large/medium/small frames or athletes/couch potatoes. So, take what it says with a grain of salt. Because I am tall and have a small frame, I barely make the cutoff for being normal on the low end. Because Russ isn't as tall and carries a lot of muscle mass, he barely makes the cutoff for being normal on the top end.

Another thing to consider is that the normal range is huge! For someone of my height (about 5'8.5"), the normal weight range is 41 pounds. That is a lot of weight! There have been conversations among the experts that the cutoff for healthy should be a BMI of 22.5. Based on that number, 80% or more of Americans are at an unhealthy weight.

There are others who argue that the normal range should be moved upwards because what is normal is trending upwards. However, we think that is ridiculous. Playing with the numbers and lying to people isn't going to make them healthier. It's just going to obscure the facts.

MetLife Weight Formula

This is the formula I have always (well as long as I can remember) used for figuring out ideal weight. I don't really remember where I first learned about it as a teenager and I didn't know it was the MetLife Formula until I started doing research about health and longevity nutrition. Many people calculate their "ideal weight" using this formula and freak out that they would look like a skeleton at the weight it spits out for them. But MetLife is a life insurance company. It is in their best interest (for profit margin) to have really good data for the weight at which people are most likely to live the longest. We are not saying this number has to be your weight goal. We are just putting the data out there for your consideration. Here's how it works:

Women with a medium frame (how to determine your frame is below):

Start with 100 pounds. Add five pounds for every inch above 5 feet in height.

Example: a medium-framed woman who is 5′5″ would have an ideal weight of 125 pounds (MetLife now provides tables with ranges rather than expecting people to do the calculation. The most recent tables, from 1984, show a range of 127-141 pounds for a woman of this size).

Men with a medium frame:

Start with 106 pounds. Add six pounds for every inch above 5 feet in height.

Example: a medium-framed man who is 5′11″ would have an ideal weight of 172 pounds (MetLife tables say the range is 154-166 pounds).

Variation +/- up to 10% for large or small frames. Frame size is determined by encircling your wrist with your thumb and first finger. If they touch: medium frame. If there is a gap: large frame. If they overlap: small frame. This isn't exact science, but it will give you a general idea.

Using this formula, my ideal weight would be 128.25 pounds (keep in mind I have a small frame).

Fuhrman Longevity Formula

Dr. Joel Fuhrman, author of the book Eat to Live and the creator of the Aggregate Nutrient Density Index, has a slightly different calculation:

Women: Start with 95 pounds and add four pounds for every inch over 5 feet in height.

Example: A woman who is 5′5″ would have an ideal weight of 115 pounds.

Using this formula, my ideal weight is 129 pounds.

Men: Start with 100 pounds and add five pounds for every inch over 5 feet in height.

Example: A man who is 5′11″ would have an ideal weight of 155 pounds.

Interestingly, in searching Dr. Fuhrman's current website there is no mention of his formula or information about if he allows for variation for different size frames. His calculation is about 10% less than the Met Life formula, meaning it lines up their small-frame allowance.

Waist-to-height ratio

A 2012 study found that keeping your waist circumference at less than half of your height can help increase life expectancy. So, our 5′5″ woman would ideally have a waist measurement less than 32.5″ and our 5′11″ man would have a waist measurement less than 35.5″ They don't provide a bottom number so it doesn't help us much with the "you're too thin" issue.

As mentioned above, we are NOT sharing this information so you can start judging yourself by an ideal number calculated by any of these methods. We are sharing it because as you start providing your body with the nutrients you need and reducing the processed food stuffs you've been programed to eat by the food industry, your body will start heading towards its ideal weight. As you approach it, the people in your life might start worrying about you. Having the data points to share so they can stop being concerned (nagging, judging, annoying) might prove to be as helpful for you as they are for us and our clients.

Helpful Science Basics

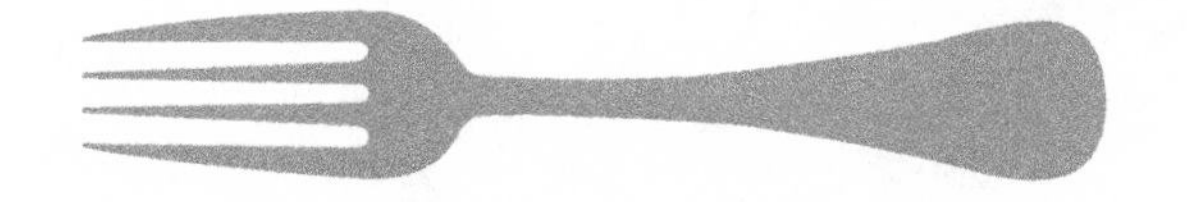

This section is a high-level summary of some of the most convincing science that led us to start eating the Whole Food Muscle Way and why our clients decide it's the right choice for them. If you're like me, you'll want to read all of it carefully and take notes. If you're like Russ, you'll read the chapters that seem relevant to you. And if you're like many of our clients, you'll decide you want to just jump in to starting the Whole Food Muscle Way and you'll skip to that section starting with chapter twenty-four.

Whichever choice is right for you is perfect.

The Protein Cult

"But how do you get protein?" If we've heard that question once, we've heard it a hundred times. It was one of the first questions Russ asked when we started researching this way of eating. But it's not something you have to worry about.

You don't need NEARLY the amount of protein you think you do. We don't care how much time you spend in the gym, how much bulk you're trying to add or if you're trying to shred. If you are guzzling protein shakes, eating protein bars and using every excuse to take in more protein, you're getting too much! If you are eating the Standard American Diet, or anything close to it, you are getting too much. Let us say that again for the people in the back – You are taking in TOO MUCH PROTEIN! And that's not a good thing. It's not even a neutral thing. It's a bad thing.

What is protein?

There is only one multicell-organism on the planet that doesn't contain protein – mistletoe. So other than single-celled beings and one parasite, protein is in every living thing. Protein is made up of amino acids, essential, which means we can't make them ourselves, and nonessential, that we can make. Amino acids are the building blocks of human cells.

The rise of a single, animal-based macronutrient

If you look at pictures prior to about 1950, you would see very few overweight people and almost no one was obese. So much so that being overweight was thought of as a good thing; it would tip the odds in your favor that you would survive an infectious disease outbreak. Only the very wealthy were overweight and suffered from the metabolic diseases that kill so many today because they could afford to eat meat every day. For most, meat was used sparingly to add flavor. There might be a bite or two and the rest of the plate was filled with vegetables and starches. On special occasions, there might be roast beef or chicken.

Meat, milk and eggs became such prized source of calories that governments started subsidizing them. Pretty soon, not only the rich could afford them – saturated fat and cholesterol for all! Unfortunately, much of Western medicine behaves as if we are all malnourished and need more meat on our bones so we can survive the next epidemic. Newsflash – most of us are dying of metabolic diseases and the only epidemic we are suffering from is the obesity epidemic!

Why animal protein is considered better

In 1914 two scientists at Yale University did a study looking at how well rat pups grew eating animal protein versus plant protein. They discovered that rat babies don't grow as well eating only plants. From there, they made the large leap to saying animal protein was also better for humans. And since the human body can process animal protein more efficiently (more easily is not better in this case) than it can plant protein, animal-based protein was given Class A status and plants, Class B. The higher biological value or ease of processing came to mean "high-quality."

What they failed to observe in 1914 and has been steadfastly ignored since is milk from mommy rats has ten times the protein as human breast milk because rats grow ten times faster than humans. Does that mean we should feed human babies rat milk if we want them to grow better and faster? Clearly there is a flaw in the logic.

Even though their assumption that animal protein was better for humans was incorrect, it has stuck for more than 100 years!

The fallacy of complete protein

Plant proteins have been labeled "incomplete" because their amino acid profile does not match that of human flesh. If humans wanted to match their amino acid profile exactly, they'd have to eat other humans (Ewww!). Plant proteins are not incomplete when it comes to fulfilling our dietary needs. Think of amino acids (protein) like a beaded necklace. Each color bead represents a different amino acid. The human body takes the necklace apart, regardless of the order of the beads, and puts it back together in the order it needs.

So where did this idea of humans needing complete proteins come from? In 1954 nutritionist Adelle Davis wrote a book called Let's Eat Right to Keep Fit in which she suggested the idea of combining plant proteins. Then, in a 1975 Vogue magazine (because they are experts in nutrition?) published an article that suggested humans needed to get all the essential amino acids at the same time to be healthy. They shared the concept of combining plant foods like beans and corn or wheat.

While you certainly CAN eat beans with corn or wheat, you don't HAVE to. Your body isn't so dumb as to need all the building blocks at the exactly the same time. Imagine what a mess it would have been in human evolution if we had needed an exact type and quantity of specific amino acids at every meal.

Side note: If anyone has the February issue of Vogue from 1975, we would love to see the references they used.

How protein really works

The human body has two sources for amino acids if it needs them and you didn't eat that one in your last meal. The first is the old proteins in your body, which is a "complete" protein because you built it yourself. Human cells aren't static. They wear out and get replaced. Those building blocks aren't just sent to the trash. They are recycled into new cells. Because your body is made up of all the essential amino acids (just like any animal flesh), you have a magic recycling plant pumping out any amino acid you might need at the moment.

The second source is a store of free amino acids just hanging around waiting to be used. Not all the protein you eat is used instantly. Your body keeps some amino acids in reserve for when you need them.

How much protein do you need?

The protein turnover in our bodies has been estimated by scientists measuring nitrogen balance (a component of protein metabolism). The Estimated Average Requirement (EAR) for protein as reported by the U.S. government is 4-5% of total calories. But since the government wants to make sure they cover everyone, they provide the RDA (Recommended Daily Allowance) which is 8-10% of total calories (RDA = EAR + 2 standard deviations covering 98% of the population for you stats nerds). Eating the Standard American Diet (SAD) will give you 15-20% protein, mostly from animal products attached to saturated fat and cholesterol. Eating the Whole Food Muscle Way provides 10-12% protein, no saturated fat or cholesterol ingestion required.

So, eating the way we do gives us twice the EAR and spot on (or just over) the RDA. We think that works out pretty well.

On the rare occasions when someone needs more than 10% of their calories to be protein, this is easily done by increasing legumes, nuts and seeds.

Animal protein is not optimal

When we eat out and the server asks, "Do you want to add protein to your salad?" I will often respond, "Sure. What type of beans do you have? Or maybe tofu?" It always results in a blank stare. Only animal flesh is considered protein in the restaurant industry.

But animal protein not only comes with saturated fat and cholesterol which lead to obesity, heart disease and type 2 diabetes. It brings other problems connected to cancer.

IGF1 (Insulin-like growth factor 1) – Ingesting animal protein raises IGF1 in humans and is linked to cancer cell growth and inhibiting cell death which is the natural process our bodies use to repair and replace worn out cells. Combining these two factors helps cancer spread aggressively. Ingesting milk in any form (whole, skim, cheese, cream, etc.) regardless of species (cows, sheep, goats, etc.) has IGF1 in it naturally (even more if it's not organic) to help baby animals grow. In cattle, that baby is 100-ish pounds at birth and grows to 400-ish pounds in about six months. Your body does not need that kind of growth factor.

Heterocyclic amines (HCAs) – When animal protein is cooked, particularly over an open flame or at high temperatures (we are looking at YOU frying, grilling, barbecuing and smoking), HCAs form. The evidence is the charring or burning of the meat. Lab studies have linked

HCAs to malignant cancer growth and human trials have confirmed the correlation. Of course, correlation doesn't mean causation, but is it really worth the risk?

TMAO (trimethylamine-N-oxide) – TMAO is a compound created by human gut bacteria when it digests the lecithin and carnitine in animal proteins (specifically eggs, poultry, dairy, liver, red meat, pork, duck, lamb, venison, fish and shell fish). Research at the Cleveland Clinic has shown that levels of TMAO in the blood can predict risk for heart attack, stroke and even death. Want to reduce TMAO in your blood? Get your protein from plants.

Acidosis (too much acid in the blood) – Let's recall that protein is made up of amino ACIDS. When our body becomes overly acidic, called metabolic acidosis, it goes into panic mode to bring our blood pH back into range and keep us alive. Acid is offset by using the calcium from our muscles. Over time this can cause our muscles to waste away. It has even been suggested that muscle loss as we age isn't a given; it's caused by our almost constant state of low-grade acidity. Fortunately, eating the Whole Food Muscle Way is alkaline and therefore does not create an acidic state.

Lab studies have linked HCAs to malignant cancer growth and human trials have confirmed the correlation. Of course, correlation doesn't mean causation, but is it really worth the risk?

Is it possible to take in too much protein?

If you are eating animal protein, it is very easy to exceed the 8-10% of calories your body needs from protein. One eight-ounce burger has all the protein you need for the day, plus fat and cholesterol you don't need. Once your system is "full" of protein, your body has to process and eliminate it. Protein is not stored and is difficult to turn to fat. On the surface that sounds good. Extra protein just gets flushed through. However, the process of eliminating excess animal protein is very hard on your system. Your kidneys will be under the most strain (due to the acid load mentioned above), going into hyperfiltration mode. This is such a well-known fact that restricting animal protein is traditionally recommended to those with chronic kidney disease to reduce kidney stress.

If we know that animal protein causes kidney stress, leading to kidney function decline as we age, why are we waiting until our kidneys start to fail to reduce intake?

Fortunately, getting excess protein while eating the Whole Food Muscle Way is unlikely and plant protein, even in excess, doesn't create the same stress on the body.

Yes, you can get all the protein you need from plants

All plants have protein and eating the Whole Food Muscle Way means you get about two times the daily requirement of protein your body needs to function. If you are ingesting enough whole-plant food calories, it is impossible to not get enough protein. Unless you are anorexic or malnourished, you cannot be protein-deficient.

In 2009, the American Dietary Association said, "Plant sources of protein alone can provide adequate amounts of essential amino acids if a variety of plant foods are consumed and energy needs are met."

Some of the top contenders for plant protein: lentils (beans / peas), seeds (hemp / chia / flax), grains (kamut / barley / oats), nuts (walnuts / almonds / cashews) and nutritional yeast (add it on anything you'd usually put cheese on).

There is really no reason to worry about protein. Just eat a variety of plant foods. Being protein deficient isn't a thing. As Dr. Esselstyn pointed out, if protein deficiency was a risk, hospitals would be full of vegans rather than obese people. We are sure that in your busy life you have more important things to worry about than a myth made up by jumping to conclusions from a study of baby rats and reading Vogue magazine.

Carbs are NOT the Devil

During our Q&A after speaking engagements someone often incredulously asks, "You eat carbs?!?!" To which we respond, "Yes, whole-plant carbs make up about 80% of our calorie intake." (The rest is protein and fat split about evenly, that we get in whole-plant packages with carbs). The follow-up question is often, "Did you gain weight before you starting losing?" and our answer is "No. We both started dropping weight right away."

How did carbs get such a bad reputation? Why are people so afraid of them?

The easiest lie to believe is one that has a little bit of truth.

"Carbs" is a SUPER broad term. It covers everything from sweet potatoes and grains to cakes and cookies (which contain more fat than carbs). Obviously, those things should not be lumped together, but they often are. Processed carbs have been milled down, had the fiber and nutrients removed and then mixed with salt, sugar (a processed carb itself) and fat. Obviously, those carbs aren't actually food, and we'd all do well to avoid them.

In contrast, whole-plant starches, fruits, vegetables, grains and legumes are loaded with nutrients, vitamins, antioxidants, minerals and fiber. The vast majority of plants don't contain saturated fat (coconut being an odd exception) and our bodies can burn them cleanly. Humans have been living on these types of food for millennia. They give us the best chance to live long healthy lives. There is zero reason to be afraid of them.

So just to be clear, when we say we eat carbs, we mean we eat whole-plant starches that contain carbohydrates, not white bread and table sugar.

How did all carbs become evil?

That is an interesting question. The logic worked like this.

1. Assumption: Insulin is bad (an incorrect assumption. But let's not let the fact get in our way.)

2. Truth: Carbs raise insulin. This is how the body is supposed to work. All food raises insulin. Cheese and meat raise insulin more than pasta.

3. Leap in logic: To reduce insulin release, avoid carbs.

4. Make billions of dollars: Start with a flawed premise, add a little bit of truth and voilà! You now have a way to make money peddling complete nonsense.

So just to be clear, when we say we eat carbs, we mean we eat whole-plant starches that contain carbohydrates, not white bread and table sugar.

The average person eating the Standard American Diet (SAD) is consuming 17% protein and 35% fat, which means only 48% carbohydrates. And many of those carbs are the processed, nutritionless carbs found on store shelves in boxes. Very few are actually from whole plants. They blame the one whole-plant carbohydrate they eat, the potato, for making them fluffy. The issue is really the butter, cheese, sour cream and bacon they load on it, not to mention the slab of meat sitting next to it.

That people lose weight when they first cut carbohydrates doesn't hurt the money-making machine. That happens because they are reducing their calorie intake (stop eating the potato and you stop eating the "loaded" you were putting on it) and their body burns the glycogen (back up battery fuel) it has stored in the muscles and liver. Just burning the glycogen can account for about six pounds of weight. But weight loss alone does not equal healthy.

One big proponent of the low-carb craze claims 44% of Americans limit their carbohydrate intake as part of what they believe is a healthy diet. It's sad. They are causing damage to their bodies by limiting their nutrition and not reaching a healthy weight doing it.

On to the science.

The human body uses carbs as fuel and is really lousy at converting them to body fat. It has three ways of using carbs before converting them to fat (which is an energy-intensive process).

First, they are turned into blood glucose, which, as we mentioned before, has the unfortunate nickname of "blood sugar," which many people assume makes it bad, like table sugar. It's not. Every single one of your cells runs on glucose. No glucose, no cell function. No cell function = death.

Second, as noted above, carbohydrates are stored as glycogen in our liver and muscles to be burned when we aren't actively digesting food.

Third, your brown fat cells use carbs to create body heat.

Additionally, the brain runs exclusively on glucose, about 500 calories worth a day. Your body CAN create brain fuel from sources other than carbs. BUT we personally don't want to force our bodies to do things the hard way when it comes to our brains. Especially since carbs aren't what's making us fat anyway.

Another benefit of whole-plant carbs is that they come packaged with fiber. It fills our stomachs so our stretch receptors feel full, slows down digestion so we feel fuller longer, has amazing nutrients that only the bacteria in our gut can release and use (gotta keep those gut bacteria happy and healthy!) and grabs onto toxins dumped into the intestines by the bile duct. Fiber keeps everything moving through the system. You can't complain about that.

We also get asked, "What kind of carbs do you eat?" The short answer, "We eat ALL the plant starches." But most commonly, whole wheat bread (See Russ' Rustic Bread recipe), whole wheat pasta (make sure the ingredients say "whole wheat" and not just the front of the package), all types of potatoes, all types of sweet potatoes, kamut, barley, steel cut oatmeal, quinoa and beans in many forms (there are at least 101 different types of beans – pick one or several).

Just last week we had a client say, "I'd really like to know why I don't feel hungrier." To which we responded, "You aren't hungrier because you are eating starches which fuel your body correctly AND have fiber which creates volume to make you feel full while taking time to process."

Whole-plant carbs have a high nutrient-to-calorie density ratio (that's a good thing). When you eat this way, you will no longer have those late-night snack attacks because your body is getting the nutrients it needs. No more craving nutrients but eating empty calories!

We have been led astray by "carbophobia" propaganda. Advertising, infomercials, sales pitches, friends who lost a little weight and diet books by doctors using anecdotal stories and playing with the science to make money. Stop being scared of carbs. Go, fill up on all the whole-plant starches (scary, but true). They will make you feel full, make you healthy and move you towards your ideal body weight!

Cheese May Be the Death of You

Cheese is one of America's (and the world's) favorite foods. The ooey gooey, salty, fat is so popular it even has its own memes. The U.S. is one of the world's largest producers of cheese. And we export almost none of it (meaning we eat it ALL). Cheese in and on everything (have you noticed?). Thanks in part to the government having WAY too much of it due to subsidies and the industry realizing they can add it to basically cardboard and people will happily eat it. And of course, there is the mistaken belief that the calcium and protein in it is good for us. Most people believe cheese is a great snack, ingredient or even a meal (we used to). Except it's not any of those things.

Let's start by being clear what milk (less concentrated cheese) is supposed to do: make sure a 100-pound calf keeps coming back to eat and turns into a 400-pound animal in about six months. According to BeefTalk, calves should average a daily weight gain of two pounds during the growing season. How could anything supposed to cause that kind of weight gain in calves do anything but cause weight gain in humans, especially in a concentrated form?

How cheese makes you fat

The average American eats 33 pounds of cheese a year and almost three quarters of that is calories from fat. It is much easier for your body to store fat than use it as energy. So, if you're taking in more energy (calories) than your body needs, it will be stored on your belly, hips and even around your organs (or anywhere else your body can find to stash it). For comparison, if you eat pure sugar, your body has to turn those carbohydrate calories into fat (burning calories to do so) before it can be stored. Humans are nothing, if not efficient machines. Carbohydrates are made for burning and fat is made for storing and given the option, your body will do exactly that.

You might be thinking, "Well, I just won't take in too many calories so my body will burn the cheese and all will be merry." Sadly, no.

> *Let's start by being clear what milk (less concentrated cheese) is supposed to do: make sure a 100-pound calf keeps coming back to eat and turns into a 400-pound animal in about six months.*

Cheese and cholesterol

Cheese will raise your blood cholesterol level, but it might not do so the way you think it does. There is cholesterol in cheese. However, some studies suggest the eating cholesterol isn't what causes high cholesterol directly. The problem is that foods that are high in cholesterol are also high in saturated fat. The National Cancer Institute ranks cheese as the top source of cholesterol-raising fat in the American diet. So, it might be the saturated fat and not the cholesterol itself that is causing the rise in your cholesterol. This has led the Dairy Association to say the relationship between cheese and cholesterol is "complicated." But really, it's not. Eating cheese leads to higher blood-level cholesterol. How it does it is just semantics.

Will cheese raise insulin?

All food raises blood sugar (glucose). That's what food is supposed to do because it is what keeps our bodies alive. A raise in blood sugar causes insulin to go up because that is how the glucose is moved out of the blood and into the cells as energy. Usually carbohydrates get a bad name for raising blood sugar (Read chapter **Carbs are Not the Devil** for more on that). Cheese has a low glycemic index so you might think it doesn't spike blood sugar and thus it doesn't raise insulin. But according to an article in the British Journal of Nutrition, dairy has a disproportionately high insulin index (the pancreas secretes more insulin than you'd expect based on the glycemic index). It is thought to be caused by the protein in milk (casein and whey) rather than the fat. In short, yes cheese will raise insulin levels.

Why does cheese cause constipation?

This is another reason why eating cheese makes you "fat." It keeps your body from "taking out the trash." A healthy colon will move about one pound of poop a day. However, if you're not getting the fiber you need, things slow down, WAY down. To the tune of not pooping for more than two weeks! Obviously, that's an issue for your health and will show up on the scale. Cheese is all fat and protein and there is no fiber to help it move through the system, meaning things don't function like they should. This is another area where the industry says silly things like, "Cheese doesn't cause constipation. Lack of fiber does." That's like saying, "Putting water in your gas tank doesn't cause your car to not run. Lack of gasoline does." It should also be noted that fiber is what grabs onto the bile produced by your liver to remove toxins from your body. When the system is slow, those toxins can be reabsorbed into the blood stream. Cheese is not grabbing any bile and toxins on its slow march out.

Why is cheese addictive?

We mentioned above that cheese has a protein in it called "casein." Casein is present in all mammal milk. It turns into casomorphin, which is an opioid compound, in the stomach. It is the reason a baby relaxes and often goes to sleep after nursing. It makes them feel good and signals to the brain that they should come back for more. Really good for the survival of the baby and the species, but not so good for adults eating cheese. For reference, the protein in human milk is about 40% casein and 60% whey. Cow's milk is 80% casein and 20% whey. You can see right there why we have a problem. Now consider that the whey is removed during the cheese-making process (that "trash" is what whey protein powder is made out of). All that is left in cheese is casein protein. If casein turns into an opioid compound and the protein in cheese is straight casein, it follows that cheese has addictive characteristics. This is also very clear in the ugly backlash we get from people when we suggest cheese is not a healthy choice. It is really like trying to take drugs from an addict.

Cheese and hormones

Most milk consumed by humans comes from cows and usually pregnant cows. Consider the hormones that course through a woman's body when she's pregnant. It's no different with cows and those hormones end up in their milk and therefore in cheese. Various types of estrogen are the most common. And the further along in her pregnancy a cow is, the higher those hormones are in her milk.

But the normal cow hormones aren't the only hormone you'll find. There is also bovine growth hormone (rBST) produced by Monsanto (yes, same group that gave us Roundup) that is injected to increase milk production. If it goes into the cow, it comes out in the milk. But don't worry (sarcasm coming) Monsanto says it's safe because it's really not very much hormone. Then the cows have to be treated for the infections that are a side effect of the growth hormone, so add antibiotics.

If you buy organic cheese, at least all you're getting is pregnant cow hormones and (in theory) not the other human-added stuff.

Cheese and cancer

Maybe you're thinking, "All of that being true organic cheese in moderation can still be part of a healthy diet." (See the chapter, **Why Moderation Doesn't Work** for why that is a ridiculous thing to say.) Let's talk about what the science shows about casein and its link to cancer growth.

Dr. T. Colin Campbell did years of research in his lab at Cornell University. Studying rats, he found that cancer promotion, or growth, can be turned on and off depending on the amount of casein in the diet. 5% casein = cancer off. 20% casein = cancer on. But that was rats. Maybe it can't be generalized to humans. Dr. Campbell went on to be involved in the largest human epidemiological (incidence, distribution, and control of disease) study ever done. In summary of years and years of work: Increased animal protein (including casein) consumption = increased cancer rates. If you are interested in the details, we highly recommend his book, The China Study. (Be warned that it is a bit dense. But if you want facts, read it or listen to the audio version. It is VERY good.)

How cheese is produced

If you are convinced that cheese, and dairy in general, should not be a part of a healthy diet, you can stop reading this chapter now. If you'd like even more reasons, keep reading. But be warned, what comes next is not very appetizing.

Cheese might be the most processed "food" on the planet. It starts out as grass (hopefully, but more likely soy and/or corn and other not-plant stuff they feed cows). It goes through the cow's digestion process (being chewed, burped up and chewed again, through four stomachs) and by magic gets turned into milk. If the cow has an infection (which is pretty likely) there is also going to be puss and blood (yuck!).

It takes a gallon-plus of milk to create a pound of cheddar. A Holstein (black and white milk cow) produces about six gallons of milk a day. But since not all cows are in the same place in their milk production cycle and their current pregnancy, not all milk is created equal. Clearly the end-result cheese has to be consistent so each truck load of milk is "standardized." That means adding cream, skim milk or skim milk powder, adjusting the color (usually with a tree extract) and pasteurizing (heating to kill bacteria such as Salmonella, E. coli, and Listeria).

Now we have a pool full of milk that has been adjusted to the needed balance. We need a way to break down the proteins. Bacteria, mold or yeast are commonly added (yes, we killed bacteria with pasteurizing and now we are adding different bacteria). If you've ever smelled cheese and thought stinky feet or dirty gym bag, that's because it's the same bacteria (yes, really).

What do you think is the best way to get liquid milk to separate into liquid whey and solid curd? If you guessed the enzyme from a calf's fourth stomach, you'd be right. Sometimes they use a bacteria (yes another one) and fungi which together produce the enzyme and for softer cheeses, acids like vinegar can be used.

The whey is drained off and sold to body builders and the public who have been brainwashed to believe they need more protein in their lives

(We used to be among them. We cannot tell you how much money we spent on whey protein in the decades we used it). The casein curds are pressed into molds to remove more of the whey, allowed to age, more bacteria is added if needed, then salt is added to stop the growth of the bacteria (cheese is in the top 10 sources of sodium in the American diet) and eventually, it is wrapped up and shipped out to you as food with some serious marketing thrown in for good measure.

The final word

Cheese is clearly not a health food. It's not the source of good protein we've been led to believe. The dairy industry has its talons deep in government policy. The work by Dr. Campbell and others has been buried and smeared by the dairy industry. And even though we don't often talk about the ethical treatment of animals or the environment, things are bad on that front too.

We are often asked, "Do you miss cheese?" Sometimes, especially on a fasting day when I see videos on social media of recipes dripping in cheese, my brain says, "You know, we used to really like that." And sometimes something reminds me of the Friday evenings by the fire with Russ, a bottle of wine and blocks of cheese and I think, "That used to be fun." To say, "No, I never miss it" wouldn't be entirely true. But it's kinda like thinking about something fun you used to do with an ex. Just because you had some fun times doesn't mean you'd take your ex back.

We've laid out the truth about cheese as plainly and honestly as we can based on the vast amount of research we've done. What you choose to do with it is up to you. But we do know this: winners learn, make plans and create change before there is a crisis. Losers obliviously keep doing what they are doing, regardless of what they learn, until they can't do it anymore. Sadly, in the case of health and longevity, can't often means serious illness or death.

Cheese might be the most processed "food" on the planet.

Nuts, Seeds and Fat

When I tell someone that we eat nuts, usually pecans or almonds because I'm allergic to walnuts, they often say, "You're lucky. I could never eat those; they are so high in fat."

What strikes us as interesting is that people worry about nuts being high in fat but rarely think about the fat in cheese, beef or chicken. Why have we been warned to only eat a handful of nuts so often that it's become a "fact?" With all the research we've done, we can't find concrete information as to where that idea came from. But we have found, over and over, that eating nuts instead of other snack foods has been shown to have positive health benefits.

A serving of nuts or seeds is a quarter cup or two tablespoons of a nut butter (peanut butter, almond butter, etc. – the natural kind with just nuts and maybe salt). We eat easily that much on a daily basis (except fasting days). Yes, it's a lot of calories and certainly there is fat in them. There is also protein and carbohydrates. Cashews, for example, are about 21% protein, 25% carbs and 46% healthy fat. One serving is about 200 calories (almost as much as a whole head of cabbage).

You might be a bit skeptical, but the science says nuts are GOOD for you and clinical trials have shown they don't make you gain weight. In fact, they can cause you to LOSE weight. How is that possible?

The fat in nuts makes you feel full. Your brain knows, from years of evolutionary practice, that fat = energy. When you intake enough energy your body recognizes in the form of plants, it says, "That's enough energy and nutrients. I'm full, thanks." And because of this message, you stop eating and eat less at your next meal (dietary compensation). To be fair, if your body is used to getting empty fat (no nutritional value) like that found in processed foods and flavorings, it might have learned to ignore that feeling because it's not used to getting nutrients with fat. Which means until it relearns, you'll have to be cautious you don't eat cups and cups of nuts in a sitting. This is also a risk if you are eating salted nuts as the salt will override your body's "I'm full" data. (We eat only raw, unsalted nuts and seeds.) This dietary compensation accounts for about 70% of the calories in nuts.

We have found, over and over, that eating nuts instead of other snack foods has been shown to have positive health benefits.

Not all the calories are bioavailable. That is a fancy way of saying they can measure the calories in a lab by burning them (one calorie = the amount of energy it takes to raise the temperature of a gram of water one degree Celsius. Don't worry, your body doesn't understand what that has to do with anything either). But your body is not as efficient at extracting calories from food as a flame in a lab. About 10% of fat calories are flushed right through your system never getting a chance to land on your hips.

Nuts rev your metabolism. Unlike other foods that are high in fat (animal products, which are unhealthy fat) that slow your system down, nuts have been shown to increase the number of calories you burn. In fact, you'll burn about 11 grams of extra fat in an eight-hour period. (Shh, don't tell the drug companies. They'll try to extract it, patent it and say they created a wonder-weight-loss drug).

Nuts are loaded with nutrients. The list of all the good stuff in nuts reads like a high school chemistry textbook, so we won't bore you. But the highlights are iron, calcium and vitamin E. Bonus!

Will nuts raise cholesterol?

The short answer is, no. In fact, eating just four Brazil nuts a month has been shown to reduce cholesterol. The science on this is in the early stages. But since there is no down side to eating four nuts a month, why not try it? We eat ours on the first of every month. (In this case, more is not better. Too many Brazil nuts can cause a problem with selenium. Good for you in the right dosage, but not in high dosages.)

Nuts might make you better in the bedroom. Erectile dysfunction in men and low arousal in women are often caused by early atherosclerosis (the same thing that causes heart disease). It makes sense when you think about it. Arousal requires good blood flow. So, impaired blood flow means impaired arousal. Not to mention an early warning sign that you're headed for heart disease. Eating nuts lowers cholesterol. Lower cholesterol equals better blood flow. Better blood flow… You get the picture.

In short, eating nuts will not make you fat, may help you lose weight, will lower your cholesterol and improve your blood flow and make sex more enjoyable. If that doesn't motivate you to eat nuts and seeds, we're not sure what will!

Note – The work done by Dr. Esselstyn and Dr. Ornish using diet to reverse heart disease eliminates nuts and seeds due to their fat content. There have not been studies comparing a plant-based diet with nuts and seeds to one without nuts and seeds. If you have been diagnosed with heart disease, stick with what the science shows for sure and eliminate nuts and seeds (and avocado) from your diet.

Olives, Yes. Oil, No.

The words healthy and oil have been used together for so long it has become part of our common knowledge. But like a lot of nutrition knowledge, what we know about oil is skewed. Before we explain why oil isn't something you want to actively seek to add to your diet, let us make three points:

One – Olive oil is BETTER than butter, lard or tallow. But better does not make it healthy.

Two – We all make choices in our diet about what works and what doesn't work for us. We choose not to use oil at home. If we go out to eat, we stick to eating plants and avoiding animal products, but don't stress about the oil restaurants seem to put in everything. Where the line is for you is up to you.

Three – If you are suffering from heart disease, diabetes, obesity or any other metabolic disease that line should be as close to none as possible.

Okay. On to why oil (any oil, including extra virgin olive oil, coconut oil, avocado oil, etc.) is not a health food.

It's straight fat. Oil is the most calorie-dense food you can put in your mouth at 120 calories per tablespoon. That might not sound like much. But you'd have to walk about two miles in about 20 minutes to burn it off. And that is if you only ate one tablespoon of oil a day. Look at the nutritional guide on your oil. The number of grams in a serving and the number of grams of fat are the same number, making it 100% fat.

It's 13.8% saturated fat. Government recommendations suggest your diet be no more than 7% saturated fat. Less is better.

It's highly processed. Eat olives. They are yummy and good for you. Squeezing the oil out and throwing the fiber and prebiotics away ruins a perfectly good food.

The lining of our blood vessels doesn't like it. There is a single layer of cells inside the walls of your blood vessels called endothelial cells. Eating a fatty meal damages the endothelium (what that layer of cells is called) and makes your blood vessels stiff for about six hours. Do that three times a day and your blood vessels are permanently stiff, which makes your heart work harder.

The pushback we get when we suggest oil isn't a health food is, "But the Mediterranean diet is healthy…" The Mediterranean diet is healthier than the Standard American Diet (that's really not hard to achieve). That does not make it the optimum diet for humans. AND the health factor in the Mediterranean diet is the added fruits and vegetables, not the olive oil and red wine.

Now you might be thinking, "How do I cook without oil?" You can sauté veggies in vegetable broth, sherry, water, or even their own juices. Just keep an eye on them and add more liquid if need be and they won't burn.

So, is olive oil bad for you? There is certainly science that suggests that. Does that mean you should NEVER have it? That's up to you. We choose to avoid it and all other oils as much as possible.

Ten Ways to Sneak in Your Greens

If you had a mother, you already know greens are good for you (kale, spinach, lettuce, Swiss chard, cabbage, etc.). They help with things like heart health, sexual function, diabetes, blood pressure, breast cancer, glaucoma and even depression. But if you can't get them into your belly, they are useless. We eat them raw in salad and add them to soups. But we know that doesn't work for a lot of people. So, we started asking people how they eat their greens. Here's what we learned:

Use it in place of tortillas to make a wrap. Okay, this is still raw so if you don't like dark green salads, this isn't a great option. But you could do it with lettuce to get in some greens where there aren't any.

Put it in a wrap or on a sandwich. You can do this with either raw or cooked greens and the flavor will just melt away into the other flavors.

Cook it in bean taco/burrito mix. When I make tacos, I usually sauté (without oil) onions, peppers, mushrooms and garlic before I add beans and taco seasoning. Add greens to the veggies and put the lid on it to let them steam in the juices. With the seasoning, you'll likely not even taste the greens are there.

Add it to pasta sauce and chili. You can do this if you're using store-bought or making your own. Just throw in a few handfuls and let it cook down. The acid from the tomatoes will eliminate any bitterness in the greens.

Put it in soups, stews, shepherd's pie and sweet potato lasagna. If you are making anything that requires putting veggies together and cooking them, add greens. It ups the nutrient value and you won't even notice them.

Put it in smoothies. We don't recommend drinking your calories in general because chewing food is part of the digestion process and allows our brains to realize we are full. But, if you're making a smoothie, throw some greens in.

Sauté/stir-fry it (in water or veggie broth). Use your favorite flavor. Soy sauce, balsamic vinegar or tahini are good options. Our "Fat-Free Asian Dressing" recipe in the recipe section is good on cooked or raw greens.

Steam it. Add whatever spices or other veggies you like. Pepper, nutmeg, ginger, apple cider vinegar, rosemary, dill… Try whatever strikes your fancy. We like onions, garlic and mushrooms with ginger.

Add it to hummus and guacamole. If you have looked at our "About That Much Hummus" recipe in the recipe section you know I put a good bit of parsley in hummus (yes, parsley counts as a green). You can do this with ALL the other greens as well. Spinach will make guacamole a beautiful bright green. Give it a shot. Add some greens to your next batch. Next time add a little more.

Massage it. Yes, this is really a thing. Add a pinch of salt and break down the fibers in the greens (often done with kale). We've never done it, but there are lots of people who swear it makes greens less bitter (we don't think they are bitter to begin with). I'm not sure if it's the massaging or the salt, but if that will get you to eat more greens, massage away.

There it is — Ten ways to add greens to your diet. Now go out and get yourself some chlorophyll! (The stuff that makes plants green)

As a side note: humans are not rabbits. We cannot live by greens alone. They are a great source of nutrients and vitamins, but you need starch/carbohydrates as well. Don't try to go on an all-greens diet to lose weight. It will not work and it will make you miserable.

Artificial Sweeteners are Damaging Your Gut

When artificial sweeteners first came out they were thought to be a panacea; all of the sweet enjoyment, none of the calorie guilt. What the public wasn't told was that they were known to cause migraines in people who are susceptible. The argument was we have to balance the "small" risk of migraines against the obesity epidemic. Artificial sweeteners were touted as the solution we needed. As you've likely noticed, it didn't work out that way. In fact, obesity is worse than ever. And while studies funded by the industry haven't found adverse side effects, 90% of independent studies have.

A few issues to consider:

- Artificial sweeteners are not digested, but they have been found to raise insulin. Because they aren't digested, they end up in the large intestine and negatively affect the microbiome, which raises insulin. Artificially raising insulin wreaks havoc on our body's delicate balance.

- Government approval of sucralose (made from table sugar by replacing three hydrogen-oxygen groups with chlorine atoms and sold as Splenda in the U.S.) has been correlated with a doubling of the number of cases of Irritable Bowel Syndrome (IBS) and Crohn's disease. While correlation isn't causation, it is worth noting that this has held steady across all of the countries who have approved sucralose for human consumption. If you have gut issues, eliminating artificial sugar might be worth trying for this reason alone.

- Aspartame (Made from the feces of genetically modified E. coli bacteria. We wish we were making this up.) Sold as NutraSweet and Equal in the U.S. and used in many diet drinks, turns into formaldehyde in the human body. The industry and the government say a small amount won't really hurt you. But overtime it has been shown to damage the neurological and immune systems. The concern is what is considered a "small" amount? Is that a one-time measurement or a "small" amount every day over a lifetime?

- Stevia (Made from the stevia leaf by isolating and concentrating the sweetness using heat and chemicals.) Sold as Truvia and SweetLeaf in the U.S., in high doses it causes mutagenic gene damage (a fancy way of saying it causes your cells to replicate incorrectly). If you stick with two (or less) stevia sweetened drinks a day it can be considered harmless. (We won't be using it.)

- Artificial sweeteners taste sweeter than real sugar (up to 300X) tricking the human brain into thinking it is taking in calories. When those calories don't materialize, we are more likely to overeat later.

The use of chemicals to avoid calories isn't a healthy choice. The human body can process sugar calories (honey, agave and maple syrup act the same way), but table sugar has zero nutritional value. If you need a sweetener, try date sugar (made from drying whole dates) and blackstrap molasses (a by-product of making table sugar) which at least provide some nutrients with the calories.

Full disclosure: We have local honey, maple syrup and table sugar in the house. I use honey in my tea on occasion and maple syrup in a few recipes. The table sugar is left from before we switched to this way of eating. I see no reason to throw it out. Occasionally having a treat sweetened with something your body can actually process isn't a huge deal as long as you know you're taking in sugar and making the choice consciously. The issue with sugar in the Standard American Diet is the VAST quantities of it many people ingest.

Probiotics – Useful or Wasteful?

Prior to learning about eating the Whole Food Muscle Way, I had chronic issues with my gut. I told my doctor several times that I felt like my GI tract just "wasn't working anymore." I was bloated (to the point of looking second trimester pregnant) more often than not and my gut just generally hurt. I tried everything. I took daily probiotics and a fiber supplement, which was recommended by my doctor, pills for lactose intolerance, laxatives, antacids and just about anything else I could find that claimed to help with GI issues. Nothing worked. If I ate, I was miserable.

But when we started shifting our diet towards eating more plants, I noticed an interesting pattern. When we ate plants, I would feel better. When we ate animal products, I would go back to being miserable. I stopped taking everything but the probiotics and the fiber supplement. The pattern remained. It was with some trepidation that I then decided to stop taking the probiotics. Again, nothing changed. Eat plants and everything was good. Indulge in meat products and… Not good!

When our diet was about 85% plants, I got brave and decided to wean myself off of the fiber supplement. I was pleasantly surprised. My plumbing worked fine, as long as I didn't try to put cheese through it (that was the only animal product we were still eating). It didn't take me long to decide that my gut bacteria REALLY wanted me to eat plants.

Where do probiotics come from?

Babies are born with a sterile gut. Those born vaginally pick up their first probiotic (bacteria) from their mom on the way out. However, those born via C-section get their first probiotics from the hands and clothing of the hospital staff who handle them. It should come as no surprise that vaginally born babies have a better start to their gut flora. Also, breast-fed babies have healthier guts than formula-fed babies.

While it's true, how you were born makes a difference, you have A LOT of control over how healthy your gut is based on the food you eat.

Where are probiotics in the body?

Probiotics – gut flora or gut bacteria – live mostly in your large intestine/colon.

What are probiotics?

Good, helpful bacteria and yeast that help with metabolic function.

What do probiotics do?

Our gut bacteria are responsible for several things that maintain overall health. Among them, making some vitamins and turning fiber into short-chain fats that feed our gut wall and support our immune system.

Are probiotic supplements worth taking?

We don't recommend it. For one, for a probiotic supplement to be useful, it has to live through your stomach acid and small intestine. Both of which are designed to be a strong defense against outside invaders.

Secondly, all of the available literature on probiotic supplements was done by or funded by the supplement industry. That means there is a large publication bias. They only share the studies whose findings are good for business and the current literature can't speak to safety.

One study that was done testing the use of probiotics to treat pancreatitis (it worked in rats) actually ended up killing twice as many participants as the placebo. So, while it used to be thought that probiotics at worst were a waste of money, there is now some evidence that they might be harmful.

Finally, as is the case with all supplements, probiotics are not regulated. The company making money on them gets to say how safe they are, how well they work and self-police the quality.

How can you get probiotics?

If for some reason (like you had to take a strong antibiotic) your gut bacteria is in need of some help, we recommend making your own sauerkraut. It's really easy.

Chop a head of cabbage into thin slices, massage about a tablespoon of salt into it until the juices are released (the longer you massage, the more juice you'll get), pack it into a glass jar (I use a Costco-sized olive jar), place a couple of cabbage leaves (saved from the outside of the cabbage) on top and use a Zip-lock bag full of water to push it down under the liquid.

> ***When we ate plants, I would feel better. When we ate animal products, I would go back to being miserable.***

If there isn't enough liquid to cover the cabbage, add filtered water (I'm never patient enough to massage it long enough to get that much liquid).

Set the jar in a dark corner on your counter, cover with a towel (to keep the light out) and wait a couple of weeks (start tasting it at about 10 days to see how you like it). And like magic you'll have your very own yummy probiotic. Store it in the fridge to slow the souring and enjoy.

What do prebiotics do?

Prebiotics are new to the supplement game. Basically, they are the food that probiotics eat. Prebiotics are attached to fiber (found only in plants and lost if you juice). Every type of plant has a little different prebiotic in it. So, eat a variety of plants and you'll feed your assortment of gut bacteria. Taking a prebiotic supplement is unnecessary.

How your gut flora gets damaged

Taking an antibiotic will kill your gut flora. Not 100% gone, but enough to create gut issues. If you have your appendix there are some schools of thought that believe it is designed to house a tiny bit of your probiotic to be able to recolonize your colon once the onslaught is over.

Another thing that can lead to unhealthy gut bacteria is eating animal products. The bacteria required to process animal protein and fat are stronger than that needed to process plants. All your bacteria are warring for space in your large intestine. So stronger means it can become overgrown and push out the other bacteria.

That is one of the reasons switching back and forth between eating the Standard American Diet (SAD) and eating plants can cause gut distress and why some people think vegetables "don't agree" with them. It is also why we recommend our clients transition toward eating the Whole Food Muscle Way over the course of a few weeks. Doing so cold-turkey (which is funny when talking about eating plants) can cause GI distress. It is doable and your gut will recover, but many people give up before their gut bacteria adjust, thinking they can't do it. That is unfortunate for their health.

Juicing is NOT the Answer

Extracting the juice from plants or taking juice supplements is seen as an easy way to get the recommended daily allowance of fruits and veggies. But is that really a shortcut way to not eat whole food? The short answer is no. But we don't expect you to believe it just because we said so (we aren't your parents, after all). Let's look at the reasons that juicing is not going to help you as much as they say it does.

It's easy to take in lots of calories

You would never eat three carrots, two stalks of celery, a handful of kale, some parsley, two apples, a cucumber and a bit of ginger washed down with a cup and a half of water and some lemon juice in one sitting. Not that you couldn't. It might fit in your stomach. But that would BE your breakfast. Not the precursor to your breakfast. All of those plants are great things to eat. But to take in all those calories and then eat more is a mistake. Not to mention that you left all the prebiotics in the juicer.

You aren't getting ALL the nutrients

Missing fiber. You might think, "Who cares? I'll just take a fiber supplement." (Why is adding another pill or potion always the go-to answer?) A fiber supplement isn't the same thing as the fiber in whole food. The fiber found in plants has nutrients attached to it that leave with the fiber when the juice is stripped out. Those nutrients (prebiotices) feed the good bacteria in your gut. Only drinking the juice means your gut bacteria go hungry. Starve your gut bacteria and it will die, leaving room for unhealthy flora to spread. Nobody wants that.

Fiber makes us feel full. You know the stretch receptors in the human stomach have a big say when your brain decides you've had enough to eat. No fiber means no stretch. Your brain gets the message that you haven't taken in enough energy to sustain yourself and will very shortly be saying, "Hey, we are hungry!" And sadly, that often means grabbing a calorie-dense, nutrition poor snack just to quiet the hunger pangs.

Fiber slows down digestion. Processing plant fiber takes time. Your body has to break things down and sort good stuff from waste. Your stomach empties more slowly so you aren't feeling hungry 20 minutes later. That processing time keeps your blood sugar from spiking. Eating whole fruit doesn't spike your blood sugar the way just drinking juice does.

Fiber keeps things moving. We all know that fiber helps our GI tract move waste. The last thing you want is waste sitting in your gut rotting. And lack of fiber has been linked to colon cancer. People eating the Standard American Diet don't get anywhere near enough fiber (and animal products are hard for our bodies to process, anyway). "Fixing" the problem of not eating enough fruits and veggies by juicing robs you of the chance to keep your gut and your body healthy.

It used to be thought that fiber was just a bulking agent and anything would do, including plastic pellets. Now we know that plant fiber plays a HUGE role in our health. It's sad to juice and throw away SO much of the good stuff. Don't pass on the opportunity to eat whole-plant foods.

The Yes and No of Supplements

For the most part, supplements are useless, or even dangerous. But there are some supplements you will want to take, depending on your situation.

B12

We suggest that everyone, regardless of their style of eating, take a B12 supplement. Humans, like all mammals, can make B12. But it requires a specific type of bacteria found in dirty water and soil. Since we live in a very clean world where we wash our fruits and veggies and drink clean water, we don't get that bacteria. People who eat meat might get the B12 the animal made. But since many meat animals are no longer eating the grass and bugs they naturally would, they aren't getting the bacteria to make that much B12, either.

We take a 500 mg, quick dissolve tablet of Methylcobalamin B12 twice a week. Our blood work has shown our B12 levels to be great.

Vitamin D

Vitamin D isn't actually a vitamin. It is the precursor to a hormone your body makes called calcitriol. Many people believe there is Vitamin D in milk. But milk is supplemented with it (as is orange juice and all kinds of other processed foods). Mushrooms, if they are exposed to sunlight, are one of the few plants that contain vitamin D. But it is extremely unlikely any of us are going to be eating enough mushrooms to get the vitamin D we need.

Humans make vitamin D from the sun. Being outside with your arms and legs exposed for 10-20 minutes (the fairer your skin, the less time you need) three or four times a week will give you plenty of Vitamin D. Absolutely do NOT get burned!

But since we live where being outside with exposed skin isn't a viable option for several months of the year, we take 125mcg (5000 IU) of vitamin D three times a week from October to March (sometimes into April if spring is a long time coming). Because we bike ride in the warmer months and have the opportunity to be outside during the day, we make enough Vitamin D to not supplement the other months of the year.

Many people believe there is Vitamin D in milk. But milk is supplemented with it (as is orange juice and all kinds of other processed foods).

If you work in an office, are never outside with your skin exposed or always wear sunscreen, you should consider supplementing year-round. Additionally, as humans age, we become less efficient at turning sunshine into vitamin D. 75% of Americans are deficient in vitamin D. Exactly how much vitamin D you need is going to depend on your genetics, your body size, your diet, your age, how much time you spend in the sun and the time of year. A simple blood test and conversation with your doctor will tell you where your levels are and if supplementing is a good idea for you.

Fun tip – If your shadow is more than three feet long, the sun is too far away for you to make vitamin D effectively. If you have no shadow, you might be a vampire and should not be in the sun.

Calcium

As we mention in the **Cheese May be the Death of You** chapter, eating animal products increases the excretion rate of calcium as your body uses it to offset the acidity created by animal protein. Since eating the Whole Food Muscle Way is lower in animal protein (or none at all) and higher in plants that contain calcium (leafy greens, broccoli, beans, prunes, almonds and chia seeds), it's unlikely you need to take an additional supplement.

Additionally, taking a calcium supplement has not been shown to decrease hip fractures but is related to an increased risk of heart attack due to the spike of calcium in the blood (it absorbs more slowly from food).

Remember that exercise, particularly weight bearing, is directly related to bone health. See the **Example Workouts** chapter for examples of Russ' beginner exercise plans and / or schedule a consult with him to develop a plan customized to your needs by sending an email to Health@RnRJourney.com.

There is no international agreement on how much dietary calcium we need. But the body is smart about absorbing it from plants when it needs it and not when it doesn't. Eating a variety of plant foods containing calcium (dark leafy greens and hemp seeds) will meet your dietary calcium needs.

That said, if you are on a medication that actively drains calcium from your body and / or your doctor has determined that the benefits of taking a supplement outweigh the risks for you, don't stop taking it!

Supplements in general

Supplement companies look at plants, try to figure out what about them is good for us, strip it out, put it in a pill, patent it, and then make ridiculous amounts of money by convincing us we need their pill to be healthy. Why don't they just tell us the plant they it got from? Because they can't patent that and make money from it.

The problem with this is threefold, **one** – supplements are only the parts of the plant that could be identified. When you eat an apple, you get multiple times the benefit from the vitamins and nutrients combined in it than you would if you took the identifiable bits in supplement form.

Two – those identifiable bits don't end up in a pill or capsule by magic. There is a chemical process to extract them. The supplement companies will tell you their process is safe. But they are self-regulated so… Hopefully, they are.

Three – Health supplements are not regulated in any way. Too often what they claim is in a supplement isn't or it isn't even close to what it says on the package. It might be just as beneficial for you to stick your money in an envelope and mail it to the supplement companies for nothing in return.

Full disclosure – we used to take A LOT of supplements thinking, "What could it hurt?" But the more we learned, the more we realized we could get everything our bodies needed just by eating the Whole Food Muscle Way. Boy, do we wish we could have all the money back we spent on supplements over the years! Since we started eating this way and stopped taking them, we feel better than ever.

We keep reading, studying and learning. We can't update this book once it goes to press. But we do share anything new with our Whole Food Muscle Club members. Become a member to stay up to date.

If you want to join our Whole Food Muscle Club and save over 50% off the regular member fee, go to *www.WholeFoodMuscle.com/bookdiscount* for the discount price as our thanks for buying this book.

Fighting Inflammation with Food

Inflammation is a major problem causer in the human body. Irritable Bowel Syndrome, Crohn's disease, arthritis, asthma, heart disease, autism spectrum disorder, general puffiness and many other common ailments are due to chronic inflammation.

But it's not all bad. Inflammation does have a positive role in human health. It is how we defend ourselves against foreign invaders, when you get a splinter, for example. The tenderness, redness and eventual puss (if you leave it in that long) are your body's way of expelling the splinter. But when it becomes chronic (it can't expel the foreign invader), it's a problem.

There are two ways to address chronic inflammation: One – stop taking in foreign invaders (stop getting splinters). And two – ingest substances (foods or drugs) to turn down the response.

Which foreign invaders are you taking in, possibly on a daily basis? Most likely animal proteins, specifically dairy products and the worst of the worst – cheese. Also, too much omega-6 in the form of processed foods and canola oils is another culprit. Reducing, or even better, eliminating, these "splinters" will allow your body to step down from high alert and reduce the number of "troops" running around fighting foreign invaders.

Your body also creates foreign invaders in the form of free radicals. You can reduce them by taking in antioxidants and fiber. We've talked extensively about the role fiber (only found in plants) plays in removing toxins and reducing gut inflammation. Remember that fiber supplements don't create the same happy-gut benefits. Let's focus on whole foods that can blunt free radicals and help keep inflammation in check

White button mushrooms (cooked) – a cup a day has been shown to be great. We don't eat that much, but we do include mushrooms in many of our meals.

Cherries – in this case sweet cherries, like Bing, are better than tart and yellow. Fresh is best, but frozen (how we get them) is a close second.

Berries – All berries are a great option. It's one of the reasons we put berries (usually blueberries and goji berries) in our oatmeal every morning (that, and we like them). Don't forget that avocado is a berry. Make sure you scrape all the dark green fruit off of the skin. That is where the highest concentration of antioxidants is found.

Cruciferous veggies – Bring on the broccoli, broccoli sprouts, cauliflower, kale and Brussels sprouts (and many others)!

Spices – There are several spices that have been shown to have anti-inflammatory effects. Turmeric (don't forget to add a pinch of black pepper to increase the bio-availability), cloves, ginger and the herb rosemary top the list.

The first thing many of our clients notice when they start moving towards the Whole Food Muscle Way is the reduction in puffiness in their face and how quickly their gut starts to feel better. I didn't realize how miserable I really was until I no longer felt that way. And the first thing many clients notice is how good their skin starts to look. We would encourage you to give it a try. You might be shocked how much better you'll feel.

The Whole Food Muscle™ Way

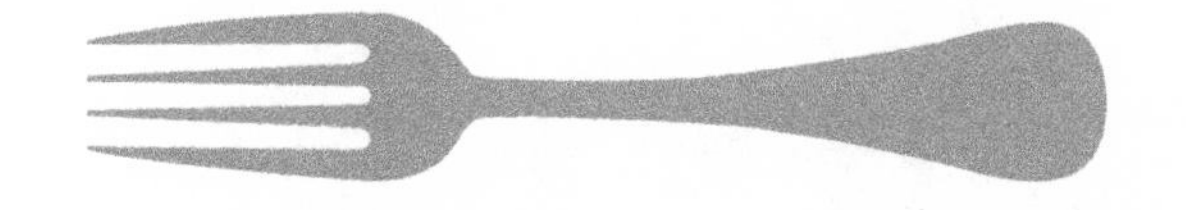

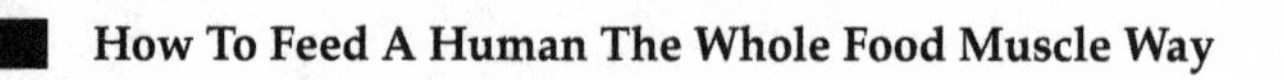

Our Journey – How we got here

Russ' journey (written by Russ)

I was teased for being chubby and wearing "husky" pants as a kid. When I was 12 or 13 years old, I subscribed to muscle and fitness magazines because I wanted to look like the guys on the cover. I started working out with a plastic-covered cement weight set from Sears. I rolled the weights out from under my bed to use them after school. I was determined to never be husky again!

As soon as I was old enough to drive, I joined a local gym. At the time the only people who really worked out were either bodybuilders (how defined and proportional can you look?) or powerlifters (how much you can lift?). The gym I joined happened to be a bodybuilders' gym. They were all friendly and helped me learn even more. I soaked up information about working out and how to eat (Everyone believed in LOTS of protein!). Before long, I became one of the most knowledgeable people there.

I competed in my first bodybuilding event at age 22. About that same time, I started playing semi-pro football. Neither of those things paid enough to pay the bills. I always had to have a "real" job as well.
Two years later I stopped playing semi-pro to focus on bodybuilding, competing in Nationals and Junior Nationals, eventually winning the Gold's Classic, New Jersey. At the ripe age of 26 and one level from going pro, I retired from competition to focus on being a full-time certified personal trainer: training bodybuilders, soccer players, football players and regular people trying to get in shape. I was also the nutritional

expert for all of my clients. As a registered trainer on the Mr. Olympia Tour, I was able to travel Europe with my client (he won the Grand Prix France, Grand Prix Germany and was the runner-up in the Mr. Olympia competition and won his second Germany Grand Prix with me as his trainer). After that tour ended, I opened a World Gym back home.

When I went to college in my mid-thirties to pursue my interest in art and design, I took athletic training and nutrition classes alongside my art, graphic design and marketing classes. After receiving my degree in fine arts and visual communication, I decided to join the "adult" world, working as a graphic designer, web designer and doing strategic marketing.

Through all of that, I worked out seven days a week and, on the side, helped people with their personal training and nutrition.

When I met Robyn in the gym, we clicked around being healthy, which for us meant working out regularly and eating what we thought was healthy. Soon our individual journeys merged into RnR Journey.

Over time, it became clear that others wanted to learn what we were doing and the Whole Food Muscle Way was born, as our way of sharing the journey with you!

If you want to join our Whole Food Muscle Club and save over 50% off the regular member fee, go to *www.WholeFoodMuscle.com/bookdiscount* for the discount price as our thanks for buying this book.

Dr Robyn's journey

Growing up on a farm, I always had a lot of energy. As a teenager, someone said to me, "I used to babysit you. I have never met a two-year-old who was so exhausting." (How do you even respond to that?) In high school I ran cross country and track but at 18, I was moved far from home and didn't have the opportunity to exercise anymore. Looking back at pictures, it's easy to see that I got a little fluffy. Not to worry though. In my early twenties I discovered volleyball, eventually playing competitively in beach tournaments. In those pictures I'm back to my lean, athletic self.

When life moved on from volleyball I continued to go to the gym and lift. But the intensity wasn't there. I no longer had a workout partner or the competitive motivation. I would go regularly, take a break and go regularly again. Sound familiar?

In my late thirties I was soft again, but not in the girlish way I was at twenty, but in a thick-around-the-middle-I-have-no-waist kinda way. When I complained about it, people would tell me I was crazy and that I was skinny. But I didn't feel it. I bought a hybrid bike (halfway between a road bike and a mountain bike) and started riding 10-20 miles at a time (weather permitting). But the weight just kept creeping on.

About the time I finished my doctorate in psychology and started my coaching and speaker training business, another nagging problem arose. My cholesterol started to do more than just creep upwards and doctors started telling me I should take a statin drug.

By 45, I was twenty-ish pounds overweight and my cholesterol hit 256. I was working out five days a week religiously (that's how I met Russ) and biking 50-100 miles a week three seasons a year. But nothing was touching my weight, which kept rising, or my cholesterol. When I complained about my chunky self to a friend she said, "Robyn, just wear Spanx like the rest of us." I tried a pair on. That was NOT happening. That could not be normal or healthy.

My doctor told me weight gain was normal as we age and suggested I see a psychologist about my body dysmorphic disorder (note – I'm the one with a doctorate in psychology. That was NOT the problem!) She was also adamant that I needed to start taking a statin.

I relented on the prescription. But, one of the side effects of taking statin drugs is muscle damage. Within six weeks of starting cholesterol-lowering medication, my shins ached so badly I couldn't sleep. I called my doctor and told her, "This is simply not going to work." She said, "Did you change your workout? Maybe it's not the prescription." But I know my body better than that. This was not overuse or injury pain. Something was really wrong. She didn't fight me on it (she knows there's no point), but she did express grave concern about my heart. Within six weeks of stopping the drug, my legs were fine and have been ever since.

It was about that time that Russ and I decided to go on what we called the "Superhero" diet. Don't look it up; it's not a real thing. We made it up. We decided we were going to eat like we thought a movie star would eat if they were getting ready to play a superhero role. For an entire month we got serious. No sauces or butter. Bread was out! Portion control was in! We had always eaten healthy (we are, after all, both former competitive athletes), so baked chicken breast, ground turkey breast or salmon with a veggie (usually broccoli or peas) was easy. And going to the gym five days a week and 20+ mile bike rides were the norm. But our weight didn't budge.

Okay then. We will just double down! But towards the end of the second month, still nothing. In fact, Russ jokes we might have gained three pounds.

It was SO disheartening! We were doing everything right but it wasn't working. We were chunky and unhealthy. And I hated looking at myself in the mirror.

We clearly were doing something wrong. Humans are not designed to get fat, suffer and die from metabolic diseases. Clearly, I needed to put on my researcher hat and find the truth myself.

RnR Journey

When we started looking for the optimal way to feed a human for health and longevity, we didn't have any expectations of what we "should" find or how it "should" work. We just wanted to know the truth about how to achieve and maintain our ideal weight and health for as long as possible. But finding information about the best way to eat for health and longevity was harder than we expected. How can so many people with Dr. in front of their names just make up stuff that isn't supported by the science? Some of them say plants are dangerous and then want to sell you hundreds of dollars' worth of supplements to make up for what you aren't getting from plants. How can there be SO many ridiculous "diets" that create weight loss, but damage your body? (We are looking at you, low-carb!)

Thousands of hours of courses, classes, certifications, continuing education credits, webinars, documentaries, books, lectures and research later we realized that eating plants was the way to go. But how do we do that? Did we REALLY need to be 100%? Was that really healthy? Russ' concern was, "What about the protein I need to maintain my muscle mass?"

We decided that trying to being 100% plant-based was more than we could expect of ourselves (how silly we were!). But we wanted to head in that direction and see what happened. Over the next few weeks we ate the meat and eggs we had in the house and didn't buy anymore. We were already eating oatmeal for breakfast. We switched out cow's milk for almond milk, started making things with beans instead of ground turkey and, because it was summer, we figured we could eat a lot of salads with chickpeas. If we had friends over or if we went out, we wouldn't worry about it. We estimate we were about 75% plant-based within a few weeks.

The first thing people noticed was my skin. Several people asked me what I was doing differently. Nothing. But then I realized, "Oh, I'm eating differently." And then the scale started creeping in the right direction.

Six weeks into our diet change, I went to see my doctor for what turned out to be just allergies (which I don't have anymore, by the way). She mentioned that she had been doing some reading about intermittent fasting and that the science seemed pretty solid. That was on a Wednesday. We got two books from the library and watched the BBC documentary Eat, Fast and Live Longer (just ignore how they eat in it) that Friday. The following Saturday was our first fasting day. (See the **Intermittent Fasting FAQs** chapter for details on how we implement IF in the Whole Food Muscle Way.) Now, the weight was steadily dropping a pound or a little more a week.

Ten weeks in, we both got our blood work done. Our cholesterol dropped 50 points each!

About three months in we had an interesting realization. We had a few friends over for dinner. They asked me to make my famous turkey tacos. Great! Easy. But Russ said he didn't want to eat turkey. Could we make beans too? Sure. A week later we ended up throwing away what was left of a pound of turkey taco meat and a container of sour cream because we weren't going to eat it. The waste was painful for me (I grew up poor, so wasting food is a no-go for me). Going forward, we decided we would just make a plant-based main meal, but still have cheese and crackers as appetizers.

A few weeks later we had different friends over. Bean tacos were a hit! And we happily ate the leftovers. BUT we had easily a pound of cheese we had put out that didn't get eaten. It sat in our fridge, taunting us, until it got moldy and had to be tossed (more waste).

It was then that we realized if we weren't willing to eat something because we thought it was bad for us, what were we doing feeding it to our friends?

About that time was also when people started noticing our weight loss and asking what we were doing, what were we eating and how could we possibly be functioning without meat? On a whim one morning I said, "We should do a Facebook Live to show people our breakfast." Surprisingly, Russ agreed (not even begrudgingly).

The first one was awful. The lighting was bad. We had really no idea what we were doing and we aren't sure anyone watched it.

The next day we did another one and it was a little better. We weren't really trying to gain anything. If it helps one person make a change toward better health, that's a win.

Then something unexpected started to happen. The more we learned (I love books, talks, lectures and documentaries about anything related to healthy eating and intermittent fasting), the more people started asking us questions. People started telling us they were creating healthy change in their lives because of the information we were sharing. We started to hear, "Can you help me? I don't know where to start."

Not being one to stray out of my lane, I decided I wanted some credentials in nutrition before I started coaching clients. I found the Center for Nutrition Studies at Cornell University and obtained their certificate in plant-based nutrition to go along with all the classes, research and reading we had been doing on our own.

At that point we had a decision to make. While it was fun to learn and fun to share, we really couldn't take additional time away from our businesses that were paying the bills, so we started to brainstorm. How do we make this viable so we can help people who are clearly so thirsty for knowledge, while still being able to pay the mortgage?

It was then that we realized if we weren't willing to eat something because we thought it was bad for us, what were we doing feeding it to our friends?

We created a survey asking our growing audience what they would find most helpful. And the Whole Food Muscle Club was born! Followed by coaching, consulting, pantry revamps, success groups, workout plans and the master class began to take shape.

And now, here you are holding our first book! We couldn't be more thrilled with our health. And to be able to share it with other high performers who are ready and willing to create their best life? That has been a dream come true!

If you want to join our Whole Food Muscle Club and save over 50% off the regular member fee, go to *www.WholeFoodMuscle.com/bookdiscount* for the discount price as our thanks for buying this book.

A Day in the Life of RnR

Weekdays:

5:00 a.m. I wake up and spend 90 minutes doing tai chi, meditation, journaling, reading and drinking water

6:00 a.m. Russ wakes up and spends 30 minutes checking the overnight stock market and news

6:30 a.m. RnR get ready for the gym

7:00 a.m. RnR leave for the gym (see the **RnR Workout Schedule** chapter for details)

9:00 a.m. RnR return from the gym (there is about 35 minutes of drive time in that two hours)

9:15 a.m. RnR do their daily Facebook Live video

9:30 a.m. RnR eat breakfast (except on fasting days)

10:15 a.m. RnR shower

10:30 a.m. RnR work

2:30 p.m. RnR eat lunch (except on fasting days), followed by a walk (weather permitting)

3:30 p.m. RnR go back to work (except on Fridays in the summer when we end our workday at 3 p.m.)

4:00 – 6:00 p.m. RnR have their fasting day meal.

Evenings: What time "evening" starts depends on our schedules, workload and the time of year. Sometimes we will work well into the evening. If we don't work, evening activities include – bike riding, going for a second walk, gardening, yard work (all weather permitting), putting together a puzzle, reading/listening to books, watching documentaries, taking online courses, playing with house plants (me), coloring (me), painting (Russ), watching sports (mostly Russ), talking/catching up with each other, local networking and corporate events.

Typically, we will eat some type of snack in the early evening consisting of fruit, nuts, seeds or other small food item. On rare occasions we go out for dinner.

8:55 p.m. "Time to unwind" alarm goes off. Yes, we really have an alarm set to remind us to stop doing what we are doing and get ready for bed. Our bedroom is our sanctuary. We have blackout shades and the bed is cozy. There is nothing we like better then ending the day kissing goodnight in our space. If your bedroom isn't your quiet place, perhaps it's time to consider adjusting that.

9:00 p.m. Bed prep – Shower, teeth, all the normal stuff. Russ also spends about 10 minutes stretching before getting into bed.

10:00 p.m. Lights out

Weekends:

Weekends are less structured. I typically get up by 7 a.m. to do sixty to ninety minutes of tai chi, meditation, journaling and reading. Most of the time Russ gets up as well. On the rare occasions he doesn't, I will crawl back in bed with him when I'm done (much more likely in the winter than in the summer).

We usually eat two meals a day, but timing depends on what is going on. Russ will always eat oatmeal as his first meal, regardless of the time of day. I am more likely to eat something else if the first meal is close to noon. However, my gut dislikes it when I don't eat oatmeal.

If we decide to have an adult beverage, Friday or Saturday evening is the most likely time to have no more than two glasses of wine.

Russ likes to eat popcorn in the late afternoon on Sundays.

Weekend activities include: bike riding, walking, yard work, gardening (weather permitting), visiting with friends, watching sports (mostly Russ), batch cooking (mostly me), doing art, doing household chores, running errands (although we often try to sneak them in during the week), reading/listening to books, watching documentaries, taking online courses and sometimes work.

It is also important to note that we both always have water nearby. We carry water bottles with us everywhere we go (I am more likely to lose mine than Russ is) and we both keep a large glass full of water near our desk while we are working. I would estimate we each drink 64 ounces of water or more a day.

RnR Workout Schedule

Exercise is an important part of a healthy life. However, you can't out-exercise a bad diet. Russ is a former competitive bodybuilder and I am a former competitive beach volleyball player. We have ALWAYS worked out (That does NOT mean we always FEEL like working out. We certainly do not. It just means we go anyway).

But all that working out wasn't enough to keep our weight and cholesterol numbers in the optimal range. Only when we changed our diet did things come in line. If you are only able to do one at first (change the way you eat or add exercise to your life), change the way you eat first. It's going to give you the most bang for your effort.

When you're ready to add exercise, this is what we do. Bear in mind that we are lifetime athletes. This is included here because we are often asked about our workouts. It is not here because we expect you to emulate us right out of the gate. In fact, please don't! Russ has created example beginner workouts for you available in the **Example Workouts** chapter. For more examples, join the Whole Food Muscle Club (*www.WholeFoodMuscle.com/bookdiscount*) or contact us Health@RnRJourney.com to schedule a personal fitness consultation with Russ.

Note: Always make sure you check with your doctor before starting any new workout routine.

Russ' Workout Schedule (written by Russ)

Here is an inside look at my current workout schedule. Keep in mind I have been working out consistently for the past 40 years. Although I no longer consider what I do in the gym to be extreme, I understand that for most folks it is. The key to any workout program is consistency. The more consistent you are, the better your results will be. Try to pick a time of day that will allow you to be consistent. For me, I like working out first thing in the morning.

My typical workout:

I do a 3-day split routine. This means it takes me three days to work out my entire body. I work two body parts twice a week and the body part that was only worked out once that week will be what I do the following Monday.

- Day 1 – back and biceps.
- Day 2 – chest, shoulders and triceps
- Day 3 – completes my whole body with legs.
- I also do alternate days for abs (abdominals) and calves and work out each twice a week.

Here are some terms for you to understand:

Reps - A rep is the number of times you perform a specific exercise.

Sets – Are the number of cycles of reps that you complete. For example, suppose you complete 15 reps of a bench press. You would say you've completed "one set of 15 reps."

Day 1. Back and Biceps (All exercises are completed by doing between 8 and 12 reps)

Back:

Lat pulldowns/pull ups - 5 sets

Standing cable rope rows - 5 sets

Standing straight-arm cable rope pull-downs - 5 sets

Seated rowing machine - 3 sets

Barbell shrugs - 3 sets

Biceps:

Seated/standing dumbbell curls or barbell curls – 5 sets

Preacher curls – 5 sets

One-arm concentration curls – 3 sets

Reverse/hammer curls – 3 sets

Wrist curls (forearms) – 3 sets

Day 2. Chest, Shoulders and Triceps (All exercises are completed by doing between 8 and 12 reps)

Chest:

Bench press – 6 or more sets

Incline press – 4 sets

Incline flies/Peck Deck – 3 sets

Cable crossovers/dips – 3 sets

Shoulders:

Shoulder press – 4 sets

Seated or standing side laterals – 4 sets

Rear dealt pull with rope – 3 sets

Upright rows – 3 sets

Triceps:

Pushdowns – 5 or more sets

Bent-over triceps cable extensions – 5 sets

One-arm over-head extensions – 3 sets

One-arm triceps concentration extensions – 3 sets

Day 3. Legs (All exercises are completed by doing between 8 and 12 reps)

Legs:

Leg extensions – 6 or more sets

Squats – 5 or more sets

Leg press – 4 sets

One-leg leg extensions – 4 sets

Leg curls – 4 sets

Alternate these two body parts. Example: I would do abs Monday and Thursday and calves Tuesday and Friday.

Abs:

Crunches – 3 sets of 20 reps

Leg raises – 3 sets of 15 reps

Weighted side crunches – 3 sets of 12 reps

Hyperextension – 3 sets of 20 reps (I always include this lower back exercise with abs. The lower back is one of the most forgotten body parts and as a result it is usually underdeveloped. This can lead to lower and upper back pain).

Calves:

Standing or seated calf raises – 4 to 8 sets

In addition to working with weights, I also incorporate 4 to 5 days a week of cardio. The type will vary between the recumbent bike, AMT (a hybrid between a stair climber and an elliptical) and treadmill. I do between 15 and 25 minutes before I lift.

Dr Robyn's workout schedule

Exercise types are just examples. Typically, each exercise consists of 4 sets of 10 reps. Actual workouts vary.

Monday:

- **15-20 minutes of tai chi**. Walks in the afternoon (weather permitting – note: Russ walks with me even if he didn't include it in his list)

- **Legs –** Walking lunges, leg extensions, leg curls, leg press, mule kicks, step ups, uneven squats, bridges.

Tuesday:

- **15-20 minutes of tai chi.** Walks in the afternoon / evening (weather permitting)

- **Chest –** Flat bench press, incline bench press, cable crossovers, peck deck

- **Shoulders –** Front and side shoulder raises

- **Triceps –** Overhead rope extensions, pushdowns, kickbacks, skull crushers, dumbbell extensions

Wednesday:

- **15-20 minutes of tai chi.** Walks in the afternoon / evening (weather permitting)

- **Cardio day –** exercise bike for an hour, outdoor bike ride for two hours or 30-60 minutes on the AMT

Thursday:

- **15-20 minutes of tai chi.** Walks in the afternoon / evening (weather permitting)

- **Back** – battle ropes, two types of pulldown exercises, two types of row exercises, reverse fly, rear delts
- **Biceps** – High cable curls, dumbbell curls, barbell curls, preacher curls

Friday:

- **15-20 minutes of tai chi.** Walks in the afternoon/evening (weather permitting)
- **Cardio day** – exercise bike for an hour, outdoor bike ride for two hours or 30-60 minutes on the AMT

Weekends:

- Weather permitting at least one bike ride of 20-30 miles, several walks, yard work, gardening (Exercise on the weekends is much more likely late spring to early fall and Russ does these things with me too.)

Send us an email at Health@RnRJourney.com to schedule a consultation to develop your personal workout goals and plan.

Exercise is an important part of a healthy life. However, you can't out-exercise a bad diet.

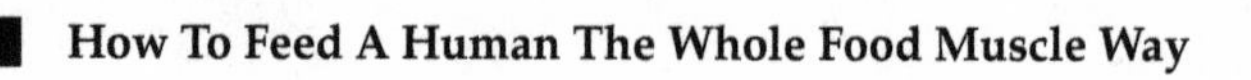

How We Eat

This is what we have found works well for us, so we always have plant-based meals available. Tweak it to your schedule's needs and food preferences.

The biggest hurdle to success is not having food in the house. Keep yourself well stocked with the staples (*visit www.HowToFeedAHuman.com/downloads* to get a copy of our staples list). You might also consider joining an "ugly food" co-op where they will send you fruits and veggies that were not pretty enough to sell at the store.

If you don't have food in the house, you can't eat it. It never occurs to us to go out to eat because there is nothing in the house. If we choose to go out, it is a conscious decision that we want to go out. And even when we do, we will often eat before we go because we like our own food better.

Meal one – We eat our first meal of the day right after our daily Facebook live (M-F 9:15 a.m. Eastern www.FB.com/RnRJourneyToHealth/). Sometimes we are even in the process of making RnR Every Day Oatmeal with fruit, seeds and spices (See the recipe in the back for details) while we are talking. Russ eats this every day (except fasting days) without fail. I eat it about 99% of the time. We like it. It's good for us. It's super filling. We don't have to think about it. Perfect!

Meal two – Russ will usually text me about 2:30 and say "Lunch?" I'd likely forget to eat until much later otherwise. We usually eat whatever main course I batch cooked during the weekend plus greens or a sweet potato with avocado and a green salad.

Snacks – Frozen fruit, fresh fruit, dried fruit, nuts, air-popped popcorn. Russ is more likely to eat between meals than I am.

Meal three – We typically don't eat a third full meal just because we aren't hungry (that is new with the Whole Food Muscle Way of eating). But most evenings we will have something light. I enjoy a tortilla or an apple with natural peanut butter and cinnamon. Almonds or pumpkin seeds are also fun to munch on.

The excuses we hear most often

"I don't like leftovers" – The biggest push back we get on the way we meal plan is, "I don't like to eat leftovers." When we ask, "Why?" there is always some story about, "My mom didn't like leftovers" or "I got sick once eating leftovers" or "I don't know; I just don't." We would encourage you to look at your reasons and see if they are valid or emotional excuses. For the record, we have never heard a valid excuse for not eating leftovers except, "I don't have a fridge." That's a different problem.

Assuming you really don't want to batch cook and eat the same one or two things throughout the week, that's fine. It simply means you are committing yourself to one of two food choices. Eat food that is prepared by someone else or cook every day. Most people who refuse to eat leftovers fall into the first camp, sadly.

There are three ways to eat food made by someone else:

- Packaged food which was made in a factory, frozen, shipped to the store, sat on the shelf, bought by you, sat in your freezer and now you're heating it up. How is that not a leftover?

- Restaurant food which is put together in a factory, partially cooked, frozen, shipped to the restaurant, put on a plate and re-thermalized (reheated) and had sauce added to it before being brought to your table. Again, how is that not a leftover?

- Someone else in your home is cooking every day.

The biggest hurdle to success is not having food in the house.

If you have someone cooking for you every day, go you. Otherwise, you are eating food that was made on some previous date and reheated. So — pretty old leftovers that are full of unhealthy stuff because it is designed to make a company money. Not batch cooking because you "don't like leftovers" is an excuse to not eat healthy food.

If you like cooking every day and have time for that, again, go you!

"I don't know how to cook" – Fortunately, cooking is a learnable skill and you don't have to unlearn all the bad habits most people pick up from cooking with animal products all their lives. If you are lucky enough to have the finances to outsource it, do that. Just make sure the person you hire is familiar with cooking in the Whole Food Muscle style, not just vegan.

"I don't like to cook" – Well, you have a few choices. Hire someone to do it. Convince someone in your home to do it for you. Get over it and do it yourself. You are a high performer. "I don't wanna" isn't really a reason to not do something you know you need to do. But you know that or you wouldn't be where you are today. People who don't do things just because they don't like them or don't feel like it don't get very far in life. That's not you.

"I don't have time to cook" – Then you certainly don't have time to be sick, feel sluggish or have low energy. High performers make time for the things that are important to them. Is your health at the top of your important things list? If not, why are you reading this book?

Bottom line

In our house, "meal planning" comes down to having lots of staples that can be used to make whatever we have a hankering for and batch cooking on the weekends so food is always available. We spend very little time thinking, "What are we going to eat?"

It is also worth noting that Russ eats pretty much whatever I cook. He doesn't fuss. He doesn't complain. He eats it because he knows it's good for him. And, fortunately, it's usually pretty good. If for some reason, there isn't enough to get us through the week, one of us will make either the Super Simple Mexican or the Easy Italian Dinner (both recipes in the **Recipes** section).

More of our recipes are available to members of the Whole Food Muscle Club. Go to *www.WholeFoodMuscle.com/bookdiscount* for the discount price as our thanks for buying this book.

What We Do When Eating Out

Without question, anything you make yourself is going to be better for you than something you get at a restaurant. They are concerned about flavor; your health isn't even part of the equation. But that doesn't mean you can never go out to eat again. How you implement eating better while eating out depends on where you are in the process. This is how we do it:

- We don't eat out often. Maybe twice a month.
- If you decide to have a mixed drink, ask about egg whites. We were devastated to learn our favorite watering hole puts raw egg whites in their margaritas (it makes them "frothy").
- We know there is going to be oil and we don't stress about it (although it often bothers our GI systems).
- We check menus online.
- We message restaurants through their website, asking about vegan options because it's easier than trying to explain no animal products including meat, seafood, eggs, dairy and oil.
- At some of our favorite places we have spoken to the manager and helped them create a vegan dish that is available upon request just by giving our name to the server (local friends even ask for it).
- Most places can do pasta in marinara sauce with roasted veggies. Just confirm they don't put butter in their sauce.
- Some chefs enjoy the opportunity to make something new. Call ahead (at a slow time) and let them know you're coming.

- Most sushi restaurants can make vegan rolls and dishes. Be aware that soups may have fish stock in them.

- If you want to have a baked potato, verify they don't rub the skins with lard or bacon fat before they bake them.

- Order veggies without butter.

- Eat before you go out. Yes, this seems silly. But we have done it when going out for social events. Particularly if it is going to be buffet style or just hors d'oeuvres.

We don't tend to frequent restaurants that advertise themselves as "vegan." We have discovered that for our tastes, they try to be too fancy with the food and too bohemian with atmosphere. We just want to eat real food made with whole plants, not faux foods designed to try and trick someone into eating plants. That said, we are sure there are other places in the country where that isn't the case. So don't be afraid to try a local vegan place.

At most places we have had good luck getting at least a vegan meal and the staff has been helpful. There have been one or two where it was a flop ("You can read the menu as well as I can. You tell me what you can eat."). If you have a place (chain or local eateries welcome) where you have had good service and a good plant-based (not junk-food vegan) meal, send us your story (Health@RnRJourney.com). We would love to hear about it!

Eating out is getting easier as more and more eateries realize there is money to be made in the vegetarian/vegan/plant-based space. The more we ask, the more the trend will spread. If you're going out, make your preferences known. It's the only way the tide will continue to turn.

When visiting friends

Some people say when friends invite you for dinner you eat what you're served. We have found that most people REALLY want to be able to serve us food that we want to eat. Sometimes they ask for recipes they can try. Sometimes they pick up a vegan dish. But usually we ask if we can bring something. We have learned when we bring a dish to make sure we get to it early because as much as people turn their noses up at eating plants, our dish is often the first empty thing on the table.

When having friends over

Early on in our transition we thought we would just eat omnivore when we invited friends. But when we stopped eating animal products because they are bad for our health, we had to ask ourselves why we would feed our friends something we knew was harming them. Now we just say to people, "Come over; we'll feed you plants!" We have yet to have anyone turn us down and everyone has enjoyed what we serve.

Try it. You might be surprised how happy your friends are to try your way of eating for an evening.

Healthy Snacking

Everyone eats snacks which are defined as munchy food (in theory, a small amount) eaten between meals. Or at least everyone wants to eat snacks. But snacking has gotten a bad rap for being an unhealthy, mindless habit that isn't good for us. And truth-be-told, the snacking industry SHOULD have a bad rap. The processed food-like substances that pass as snacks are horrible. They override our brain's ability to say, "Thanks, I've had enough" by being salt-, sugar- and fat-bombs. They have zero (or VERY close to zero) nutritional value and are ridiculously calorie-dense. So, if you're snacking on what most of the Western world considers snack food, you've got a problem; those snacks are addictive.

Why are snacks addictive?

The short answer is because they are made that way by the food industry. They spend billions of dollars determining exactly how to make a snack the right amount of crunchy, salty, sweet, and fat to make you eat the whole box/bag without realizing it. The more they can hit the "crave" center of your brain, the more money they make. And why wouldn't they? Your health is your problem. Keeping their shareholders happy is theirs.

And just for good measure, they take out any nutrients that might have been in the ingredients they used to make the product. Nutrients spoil. That's bad for shelf life. And bad for shelf life means bad for the bottom line (again, shareholders).

Will snacking cause weight gain?

If you are eating the type of snacks mentioned above, the standard ones you find in a convenience store or advertised on TV, yes, snacking will cause weight gain. BUT (this is a big but), it's not the snacking itself.

Let's break it down. If you are eating nutrient dense food during meals and you're legitimately hungry between meals, eat more! There are some days that I eat little things all day and there are some days I only eat meals. Today, I had my regular (about 1000 calorie) oatmeal at 10 a.m. Then I was hungry around noon so I had a couple of corn muffins. Now it's lunch time (2:30-ish) but I'm not hungry. So, I will likely either eat lunch later or have another small snack and then eat again when we get back from our event tonight. There is no wrong way to eat nutritious food. The key is to eat when you're hungry, not when you're bored or stressed or angry or (insert emotion or habit here). Understanding why you choose to eat what, and when is a big part of the psychology of eating and eating success.

So, no. Snacking will not cause weight gain IF (this is a big if) you are snacking on real food. But what is a real food snack?

We keep a running list of things we and our clients eat as snacks. Go to *www.HowToFeedAHuman.com/downloads* to get your copy.

So, if you're snacking on what most of the Western world considers snack food, you've got a problem; those snacks are addictive.

Staples List

One of the most common questions we get asked is, "What staples do you keep in the house?" We thought about including a list here. But that would be unfair because we are always finding new things that become staples. So instead, we created a page where you can download our current list. Visit *www.HowToFeedAHuman.com/downloads* to get started on your shopping list.

New Foods to Try

While talking to someone who has been yo-yo dieting the same 50-ish pounds for the entire 12 years I've known him, I suggested he stop dieting and start eating by moving towards eating more plants. He replied, "That's WAY too restrictive!" I explained that we eat much more variety now than we ever did on the Standard American Diet (SAD). To which he said, "You can go ahead and admit it's restrictive to me. I'm not a client."

Let's overlook the fact that he suggested we lie to our clients, and focus on the fact that it made me wonder if other people thought their diet got MORE interesting when they switched to eating plants. We have an informal survey running posing this question to the plant-based / vegan community and our clients:

"What foods do you eat now that you had never tried before you changed your way of eating?"

A few examples that have been shared with us are:

- Bean burgers
- Chia seeds
- Chickpeas
- Eggplant
- Falafel
- Kamut

- Nutritional yeast
- Turnips

For the complete list go to www.HowToFeedAHuman.com/downloads. We update it anytime someone says, "You know what I just tried?!?!" Make sure you let us know if you try something new following the Whole Food Muscle Way!

Making the Whole Food Muscle Way Work for You

1. Let go of the nonsense the food industry has created in your brain. Feeding yourself is not a hassle, a waste of time or a chore.

2. Stop relying on social media, Big Food, Big Pharma and the government to tell you what's healthy. Educate yourself with facts.

3. Let go of the idea that carbohydrates are bad and that portion control is something you have to worry about.

4. Stop worrying about protein.

5. Choose to eat 80% (or more) plants.

6. Address self-sabotage and develop grit.

7. Consider if intermittent fasting is right for you.

8. Exercise.

If your "diet" has side effects other than making you healthy and the risk you'll live longer, you're on the wrong diet.

If you would like a printable version of this list go to www.HowToFeedAHuman.com/downloads

Example Workouts

Before you begin this or any workout plan please consult with your doctor to determine if you are healthy enough to exercise.

This program is designed to tone and strengthen your entire body and improve your cardio health. If you have specific training goals, need more information or would prefer a custom workout plan, set up a one-on-one session with Russ by emailing us at Health@RnRJourney.com.

Pro tip:

The key to a successful exercise program is consistency. Pick a time of day that will work with your schedule and stay with it. We like to workout first thing in the morning. It is set in our minds that we go to the gym every morning, it's not a question. This has allowed us to be consistent for many years.

The main muscle groups:

1. Shoulders

2. Chest

3. Back

4. Biceps

5. Triceps

6. Legs

    - Quadriceps (Front of the leg above the knee)

- Hamstrings (Back of the leg above the knee)

- Calves

7. Abs (stomach)

Terms you need to know

Set – a group of reps

Rep – one movement of an exercise

Exercises:

If you are new to working out, bring this list of exercises to the gym and ask the staff to show you which machines go with which exercise. If you are comfortable using free weights, they are a great option.

Two day full-body workout

Day 1

- Bench Press (chest)
- Shoulder Press (shoulders)
- Tricep Pushdowns (triceps)
- Leg Extensions (quads)
- Calf Raises (calves)

Day 2

- Lat Pulldown (back)
- Seated Rows (back)

- Biceps Curls (biceps)
- Leg Curls (hamstrings)
- Abdominal Crunches (abs)

Start with one set of 8-10 reps of each exercise for two weeks. Weeks three and four do two sets of 8-10 reps. Thereafter do three sets of 8-10 reps. Start to increase the weight as the third set becomes easy to do. You may also increase the weight by a few pounds between sets for a bit more of a workout.

How to choose weight

Always start with light weight and work your way up to a level that is right for you. Choose a low weight and do a rep or two. If it feels like you are throwing the weight, increase the weight. Your movement should be steady and controlled. There should be some resistance but it should not be strenuous or painful.

Pro tip:

If your workout makes you completely miserable the next day or if you are sore for more than two days, you did too much. Start slowly. Doing too much too quickly will discourage you and you risk hurting yourself.

Novice example workout – If you have never worked out

- Monday – Day one of the full-body workout
- Wednesday – Day two of the full-body workout
- Friday – Twenty minutes cardio of your choice

Beginner example workout – If you've worked out in the past and are getting back into it or the workout above has become easy

- Monday – Twenty minutes cardio of your choice
- Tuesday – Day one of the full-body workout
- Wednesday – Twenty minutes cardio of your choice
- Thursday – Day two of the full-body workout
- Friday – Twenty minutes cardio of your choice

Intermediate example workout – If the workouts above are easy and you're ready to step it up

- Monday – Day one of the full-body workout and twenty minutes cardio
- Tuesday – Day two of the full-body workout
- Wednesday – Twenty minutes cardio of your choice
- Thursday – Day one of the full-body workout
- Friday – Day two of the full-body workout and twenty minutes cardio

Pro Tip:

Don't feel like you have to limit yourself to twenty minutes of cardio. If you want to do thirty or forty-five minutes, feel free to do so. As long as you are fueling your body well, cardio is great for you.

Do these workouts consistently and you will start to see a difference in your muscle tone, strength and endurance in as little as four weeks.

Recipes

We have included a few of our go-to proven recipes that we use week in and week out. For more of our recipes and my tips from about how to cook amazing meals that even omnivores will love, become a member of the Whole Food Muscle Club at *www.WholeFoodMuscle.com/bookdiscount*

Russ' Rustic Bread

- 4 cups organic whole wheat bread flour
- 2 tsp salt
- 1 tsp dry yeast
- 2 tablespoons of caraway seeds and/or everything bagel seasoning
- ~ 1/3 cup sourdough starter (optional)
- 2 ¼ cups filtered water

In a glass bowl, blend dry ingredients. Add sourdough starter (if using). Add about ½ the water and mix using a large spoon. Add remainder of water and mix until well blended. Cover with plastic wrap and set in a warm place to rise (not on granite, it's too cold and the dough won't rise) until double in size.

In the summer a few hours is long enough. In the winter it often needs to be left overnight. To speed up the rising process, place in the oven with the oven light on.

Line a 9x9 (or equivalent) Dutch oven with parchment paper. Place in oven. Preheat oven and Dutch oven to 450°. Carefully turn risen dough into hot Dutch oven (we have found the using your fingers to get the dough to release from the bowl works best, albeit messy). Score top with a damp, sharp knife if desired. Cover and bake for 30 minutes. Remove lid and bake 15 more minutes.

Remove from Dutch oven by carefully lifting using the parchment paper and allow to cool.

Enjoy with hummus, natural peanut butter or whatever (healthy item!) you love to put on bread.

Note: Wash, or at least put water in the bowl you used to let the bread rise. If you let the bits of dough dry on it you will have to soak it to get it clean.

RnR Every Day Oatmeal

Russ has eaten oatmeal basically every day for forty years. When I met him, I thought that was crazy. Now I eat oatmeal with rare exception.

- ½ cup organic steel cut oats
- ¾ cup fresh or frozen blueberries (can substitute any berries you like)
- 1 tablespoon hemp seeds
- 1 tablespoon chia seeds
- 2 tablespoons ground flaxseed
- 1 tablespoon sunflower seeds (optional)
- 1 tablespoon pumpkin seeds (optional)
- A pinch of goji berries (optional)
- ½ tsp turmeric
- ½ tsp cinnamon
- 1 tsp Alma powder (Ground Indian gooseberry. Available at *www.RnRJourney.com/store*)
- ¼ tsp Dulse flakes (Seaweed. Also available at *www.RnRJourney.com/store*)
- 1 twist of the black pepper grinder
- A handful of raisins
- 1 banana

Place oatmeal in a large bowl. Add enough water to just cover the oatmeal. Add berries. Microwave on high for 2.5 minutes. Add everything else. Stir. Add more water if it seems too dry (Add slowly. We make soup by accident every now and then). Heat for another minute or so, if desired. Enjoy.

Note: Dr Robyn uses a 1/3 cup of oatmeal, does not include the banana and is more likely to leave the sunflower seeds out.

About That Much Hummus

Here's the thing about hummus – you can't really make it wrong. There are some basic ingredients. Put them together in whatever balance works for your taste buds and then add whatever flavor you feel like having (or don't). Hummus is a wonderful spread for sandwiches, a topping for potatoes and a dip for just about everything. We eat it every day.

Starting point:

- 3-ish cups chickpeas (or any other bean you want) – I use canned because it's easy. I do rinse them. Some people swear by cooking dried beans. If I make it with something other than chickpeas, I cook my own. But as of right now, canned chickpeas are just easy. We eat A LOT of hummus. I make 3 or more cups every 4-5 days and more if we have company.

- Juice from one large lemon or two large limes – If I want more tang, I will also add the zest (Russ isn't as big a fan of this as I am).

- ½ cup tahini – Some people say this is oil because sesame seeds have oil. Leave it out if you want it oil-free.

- 2-3 chopped garlic cloves – more or less depending on how much you like garlic and how big your cloves are. Russ is Italian, so…

- Cumin, or not – I typically add a nice round tablespoon of cumin. But I ran out the other day and made it without. It was not the end of the world.

- ¼ cup parsley – Or more. I just dump some in there. Fresh is best. Dried works too.

- Add water, chickpea liquid or juice from any flavor you're using if needed for consistency

Add all to your food processor and blend. Before I had a food processor, I used the immersion blender. It required the hummus be a little thinner, but it worked.

Flavor ideas:

- Anything you feel like trying
- Roasted red pepper (we love this one)
- Caramelized onions (If you're making a sandwich spread – this is great)
- Jalapeños (use the juice too)
- Olives (again, use the juice if you really like the olive flavor)
- Crushed red pepper (spicy!)
- Lemon (add the zest!)
- Balsamic vinegar
- Avocado (this results in a really smooth and creamy end product. I usually add one regardless of what flavor I'm making)
- Garlic (just add more)
- Sundried tomato (not packed in oil if possible)
- Paprika (or any other spice)
- Mustard (pick a flavor, any flavor. Great as a spread.)
- Pine nuts

- Sesame seeds
- Cooked mushrooms
- Pumpkin and cinnamon (this was more dessert-like than I like my hummus)
- Chocolate and maple syrup (We have never made this one. But Whole Food Muscle Club members swear by it.)

How much of any of these depends on how you like it. Put some in. Try it. Add more, or don't. There is no right or wrong answer. (Although I have made it too spicy for me to eat. Russ loved it.)

Things to dip in hummus:

Hummus is super versatile. Just about any veggie, bread, cracker or tortilla can be used as a delivery method. I have even made it thinner (more liquid) and put it over pasta. Use it as a base for your veggie wraps and sandwiches in place of mayo. It even works as part of a salad. The mustard version is great anywhere you want that tang with some heft.

Super easy to make and even easier to eat! Do you have a flavor you'd love us to try? Please share! Health@RnRJourney.com

Fat-free Asian Dressing

- ½ cup rice vinegar or apple cider vinegar
- ¼ cup soy sauce
- ¼ cup (or less) maple syrup
- 1 tablespoon grated, fresh ginger (Can sub dried ginger powder. Start with 1 tsp and then add to taste)
- 1 teaspoon granulated garlic or one minced clove (add more if you like garlic-flavored sauces)

Whisk all ingredients together. Taste and adjust to your liking. Store in an air-tight container in the refrigerator. Flavors meld nicely over time. Stir before using, as the ginger tends to settle to the bottom.

This dressing is great over quinoa and veggies, cooked greens, salads and just about anywhere else you'd like a little Asian flavor.

Russ' Quick Italian Dinner

- 1 med. onion, diced
- 1 bell pepper, diced (color of your choice)
- 2-ish cups, chopped mushrooms
- 1 tsp. garlic powder (can sub a clove or two of chopped garlic)
- 1 can black beans
- 1 jar marinara sauce*
- Greens of your choice
- 10 oz. whole wheat pasta (cooked to whatever you think is "done")

Instructions:

Rinse beans. Add beans, onions, peppers, mushrooms and garlic powder in a large pot. Cover and cook over medium heat. When the veggies have cooked down enough that there is room for the sauce, add it (you can add it at the beginning if your pot is big enough). Stir to combine well. Cook until the onions and peppers are soft but not mush.

Plate over greens of your choice (the heat from the sauce and pasta will just wilt the greens nicely). Serve with nutritional yeast and hot sauce.

Be aware, for some reason this dish holds heat for a long time and will burn your mouth if you're not careful.

As is the case with all Italian dishes, this is even better as leftovers. Which can be used to make Cheater's Lasagna. (Recipe available to members of the Whole Food Muscle Club)

*Find one with little or no sugar and oil if at all possible

Super Simple Mexican

- Black beans
- Rice (brown or black)
- Salsa of your choice
- Corn (optional)
- Cooked mushrooms (optional)

Mix beans and rice in about a 1:1 ratio (and about half as much corn if using and however many mushrooms work for you, sprinkle with garlic powder if you are so inclined). Add enough salsa to create a consistency you like. Heat through and enjoy.

Eat as a burrito, taco, Buddha bowl or whatever sounds good to you.

Serve with: diced onion, avocado/guacamole, tomatoes, hummus, chopped greens (spinach, kale, parsley, cilantro, etc.), broccoli sprouts, chopped olives, diced peppers, jalapeños, any other veggies you like and hot sauce of your choice

Extra nutrients tweak: use quinoa in place of the rice, sprinkle in ground flaxseed or nutritional yeast

Robyn's Sweet Potato Lasagna

This is not hard to make, but it is time-consuming.

- 3-4 cooked sweet potatoes (I typically boil them for this recipe but you can bake them.)
- 2 bell peppers, chopped (color of your choice)
- 2 med. onions, chopped (I often do one red and one white, but whatever you have will work)
- 3-4 cloves garlic, diced (I use the food processor)
- 2-3 carrots, chopped (I use the food processor)
- 2-3 ribs celery, chopped
- 3-ish cups chopped mushrooms (more is better in my world)
- 1 cup frozen corn
- 1 cup frozen peas
- 1 cup chopped broccoli (optional)
- 2-3 handfuls of greens (your choice, I like kale)
- 24-ish oz. marinara sauce (Your choice. Make your own or store-bought*)
- A splash of unflavored, unsweetened plant milk
- Organic, whole wheat lasagna noodles
- Sliced fresh tomatoes (optional garnish)
- Parsley (optional garnish)
- One batch of cashew Cheese-ish Spread

Instructions:

Remove skins from sweet potatoes (I find this to be easiest after they are cooked and cooled enough to handle). Mash into a paste. Add a splash of plant milk if you want it a bit creamier. Set aside. (I often do this step while the veggies cook. Just don't get distracted and let the veggies burn.)

In a large pan with a lid (I use a big, deep-frying pan) cook peppers, onions, garlic, carrots, celery and mushrooms over medium heat. Sweat the veggies, covered, stirring periodically to ensure it doesn't stick, add a splash of water or veggie broth if needed. Cook until onions are translucent and mushrooms have released their juice. Uncover and allow to cook down for about five minutes (stir so it doesn't burn).

Add peas, corn and broccoli (if using). Cook until just warmed through. If you want to add no-salt seasoning or Italian spice, this is the time to do it. Sometimes I do and sometimes I don't. How much? Eh, a good sprinkle. Let's say, two tablespoons each.

If you have room in the pan you can wilt your greens in the same pan. If not, do it in a separate one.

Noodles – I have found this dish is wet enough to put the noodles in uncooked and let them cook while it bakes. Saves time and the noodles soak up the extra liquid from the veggies.

Layer it together in a deep baking pan (I have used a 9 x 11, but I really like the deep / cheap aluminum baking pans you can get at the dollar store. Deeper is better).

Assemble: Thin layer of marinara sauce. Noodles. Sweet potatoes. Veggies. Greens (if they aren't cooked together). Cheese-ish Spread –

recipe below (it will be messy to get on there. Just smear it.). Noodles. Marinara. Etc. End with marinara and Cheese-ish Spread. Sprinkle with nutritional yeast if you'd like and then add slices of tomato to make it pretty. If I'm lucky I can get three layers. But sometimes I only get two and a half. It depends how deep your pan is and how thin you are able to make your layers.

Bake covered (I use aluminum foil) for one hour at 375° plus 20 minutes uncovered. I HIGHLY recommend setting it on a cookie sheet in case it bubbles over. Should be bubbly hot. Let sit for a few minutes to set before cutting.

Sprinkle with fresh parsley and serve with hot sauce (that's a Russ thing).

This might be a bit wetter than traditional lasagna and might not be plate-pretty. But I have served it to people who eat the Whole Food Muscle Way and to omnivore friends alike. Everyone has loved it.

As with all Italian dishes, this is even better the next day. If making a day ahead, add 15-20 minutes to bake time to make up for it being cold from the fridge. Because this is so wet, it's pretty hard to burn unless you forget about it. It can be frozen before baking (just make sure there is room in the top of your pan for it to expand a bit). I have always let it thaw before cooking. I would not go straight from freezer to oven.

If you have leftover veggies, sweet potato and/or marinara, they are really good over quinoa or elbow pasta (which is the cheaters way to get the lasagna flavors without having to do the layering bit).

*If using store bought marinara, look for one with as few ingredients as possible and without oil or sugar.

Robyn's Cheese-ish Spread

Note – this is NOT going to taste like oily, fatty, salty dairy cheese or oily, fake vegan cheese. It is meant to be used in recipes like sweet potato lasagna to add depth of flavor and mouth-feel. After your taste buds switch from the Standard American Diet to the Whole Food Muscle Way, you may like it on sandwiches and in wraps. If you have Standard American Diet taste buds, this is not "cheese." That doesn't mean you won't like it. I just don't want you to be disappointed.

- 2 cups soaked cashews*
- 1 avocado
- 1 overly ripe apple, chopped or ¼ cup unsweetened apple sauce (can get away without but is better with)
- 4 rounded tablespoons nutritional yeast
- ¼ cup lime or lemon juice (fresh-squeezed if possible)
- Salt/pepper to taste
- ¼ cup water or veggie broth

Place all ingredients except water/veggie broth in a food processor or high-speed blender (you might need more liquid if using a blender). Blend until smooth, adding water/veggie broth if needed. Taste and adjust flavor. Add other spices for additional flavor if desired. We have enjoyed Cajun, cayenne pepper, and lemon pepper seasoning.

*Soaking the cashews overnight will give you a creamier end result. If you don't have time for that, you can soak them in boiling water for 20 minutes or use them dry. You will just end up with something that has a texture similar to ground nuts (which you won't even notice if you're using it in a cooked dish). I have subbed almonds in a pinch.

Additional note – this makes a large batch created to put in sweet potato lasagna. Halve the recipe for a smaller quantity (obviously).

Thank You for Reading Our Book!

This book has not been written for everybody. It is meant to reach the top 1% of people who are high-achievers and to make the other 99% wonder how you got so lucky to be where you are.

We didn't put it together to impress you with a fancy book cover or glossy information. We wanted to give you real life, hard-hitting, practical techniques, strategies, advice, principles and real-world experience from people who have been in your shoes and share your journey.

One secret that you will uncover is, as you begin living your life the Whole Food Muscle Way, new doors will open to you. You will see things differently. You will feel better and you will look better. You may even find yourself sharing these techniques and ideas with others.

I would recommend that you sit down in your favorite spot and read this book again. Don't treat it like a book you borrow from the library. Write in the margins. Take notes. Highlight it. Re-read it.

Get to work on you. When you successfully implement the Whole Food Muscle Way and it has helped you move towards your health and fitness goals, even if just one technique works for you, please email us at Health@RnRJourney.com.

We love to hear success stories and maybe we'll meet along the journey.

We look forward to hearing from you soon and seeing you in the Whole Food Muscle Club.

Until then, all the best.

RnR

Acknowledgments

We would be remiss to make you believe this book came about without the help of some amazing people. To all the plant-based researchers, doctors, practitioners and everyday people who realized the power of this way of eating and shared it so we could learn from you, thank you. To the countless people who have shared their workout and competition knowledge with us over the years, you are a part of this too. To those who were a part of the development of our professional skills (psychology for Dr Robyn and website and graphic design for Russ), this book wouldn't exist without your dedication to teaching. To everyone who reviewed a pre-release version, you made this project better by sharing your time, stories and reactions. To all of our readers and clients, past, current and future, thank you for allowing us to be a part of your journey.

There are a few people we need to call out by name. Nancy LaFever for editing prowess, Brooke Cooper and Laura Lewis for eagle-eyed proofreading and Lee Collins for marketing, coaching, consulting and pushing us (gently and otherwise) to write this book. We are proud to call each of you friend and colleague.

CPSIA information can be obtained
at www.ICGtesting.com
Printed in the USA
FFHW020633081119
56013195-61899FF